total
strength training
for women

total
strength training
for women

amazin lethi

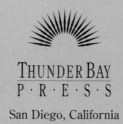

THUNDER BAY
P·R·E·S·S

San Diego, California

This book is dedicated to all those who have found the true meaning of holistic enlightenment through the world of strength training, and to my parents who have always supported me through my years as a Natural Competitive Bodybuilder.

Many thanks to Tom Henner and the Reebok Sports Club, London, for their support.

CAUTION
Never undertake any new course of exercise without first consulting a doctor. This book is meant as guidance only and if you feel any pain or discomfort with any of the exercises you should stop immediately.

Thunder Bay Press
An imprint of the Advantage Publishers Group
5880 Oberlin Drive, San Diego, CA 92121-4794
www.thunderbaybooks.com

THUNDER BAY
P·R·E·S·S

SERIES EDITOR: Karen Ball, MQ Publications
EDITORIAL DIRECTOR: Ljiljana Baird, MQ Publications
PHOTOGRAPHY: Stuart Boreham
DESIGN CONCEPT: Balley Design Associates
DESIGN: Rod Teasdale
ILLUSTRATION: Oxford Designers and Illustrators

All notations of errors or omissions should be addressed to Thunder Bay Press, Editorial Department, at the above address. All other correspondence (author inquiries, permissions) concerning the content of this book should be addressed to MQ Publications, 12 The Ivories, 6-8 Northampton Street, London N1 2HY.

ISBN 1-59223-197-7
Library of Congress Cataloging-in-Publication Data available upon request.

Printed in China

1 2 3 4 5 08 07 06 05 04

contents

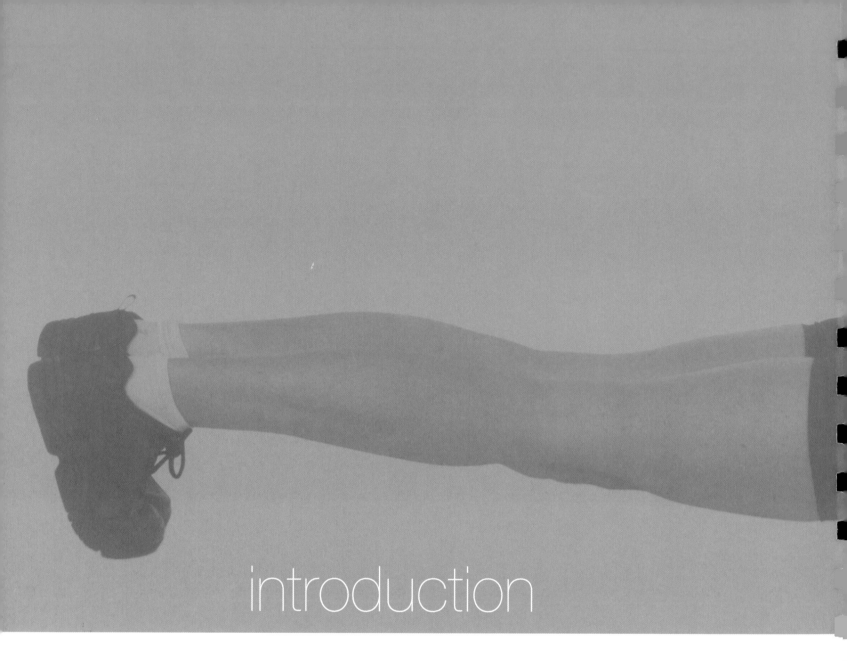

introduction

When it comes to female strength training, myths and false perceptions abound. Many women are too intimidated to even step foot into a gym, imagining a terrifying scene of unfamiliar equipment and other people's perfect bodies. Some women worry that if they do begin strength training, they might turn into muscle-bound freaks. This will not happen. Strength training is as much about toned fitness as it is about building muscle. And for any woman looking for muscle tone, weight loss, increased strength, a daily fitness routine, rehabilitation, or just overall general health and fitness, there is no better choice than lifting weights.

The intention of this book is to sort fact from fiction and allow women to enjoy one of the most satisfying and results-driven sports available. The book starts with an explanation of the basic principles and science behind strength training and discusses how to prepare yourself and what to expect as you begin training. This is followed by a step-by-step explanation of each muscle group, with descriptions of how the different muscles function and how to train them using fixed-weight and free-weight exercises that are suitable for all beginner to intermediate students. Finally, the last section of the book puts together extended routines developed with specific needs in mind.

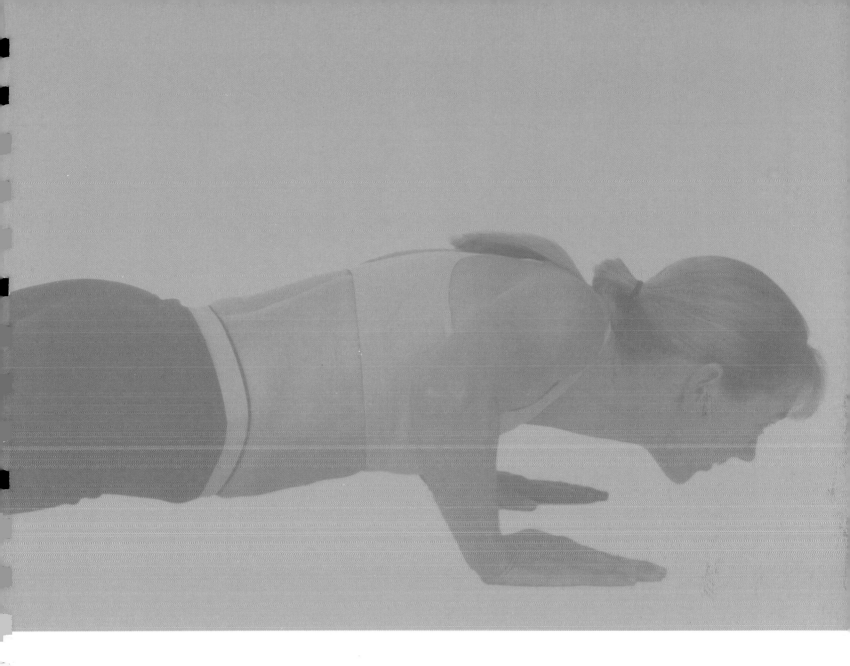

This book also provides in-depth information about training through the different stages in your life; it discusses the importance of complementary aerobic training, the differences between free weights and machines, and how the body works; it offers information on why, how, and when to stretch; and it explains the basic terms that you will come across in the world of strength training.

One of the biggest barriers to effective strength training is lack of knowledge. I have witnessed too many people train year in, year out without seeing any of the results they set out to achieve. Training without the right information will result in frustration and a belief that strength training doesn't work—which simply isn't the case. To make those weights work effectively for you, you first need to understand how to use them properly.

I started training at the age of seven and have been in the fitness industry for more than ten years, as a Natural Competitive Bodybuilder and qualified strength trainer to Olympic athletes, celebrities, competitive bodybuilders, and the general public. I know that setting realistic goals, incorporating those goals into your daily life, and understanding your own body mean that strength training really can work for you. The aim of this book is to put you on the right path to effective strength training and, hopefully, to lead you to a lifetime of enjoyment and reward.

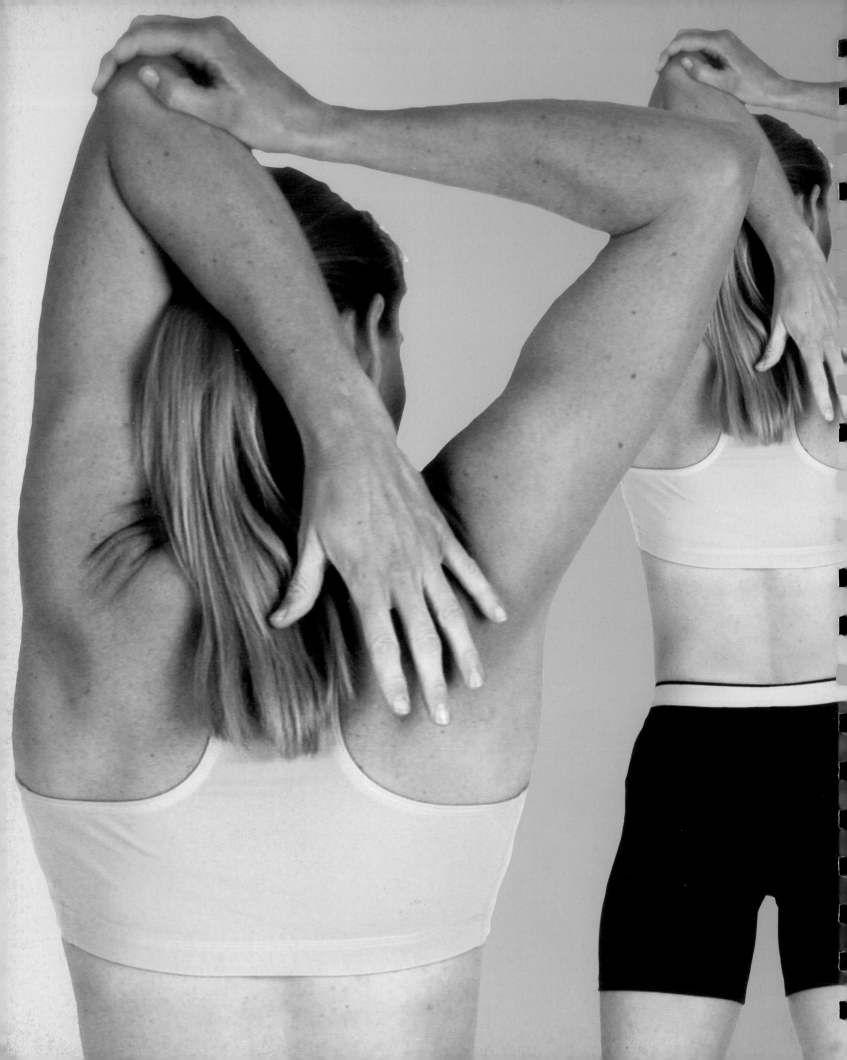

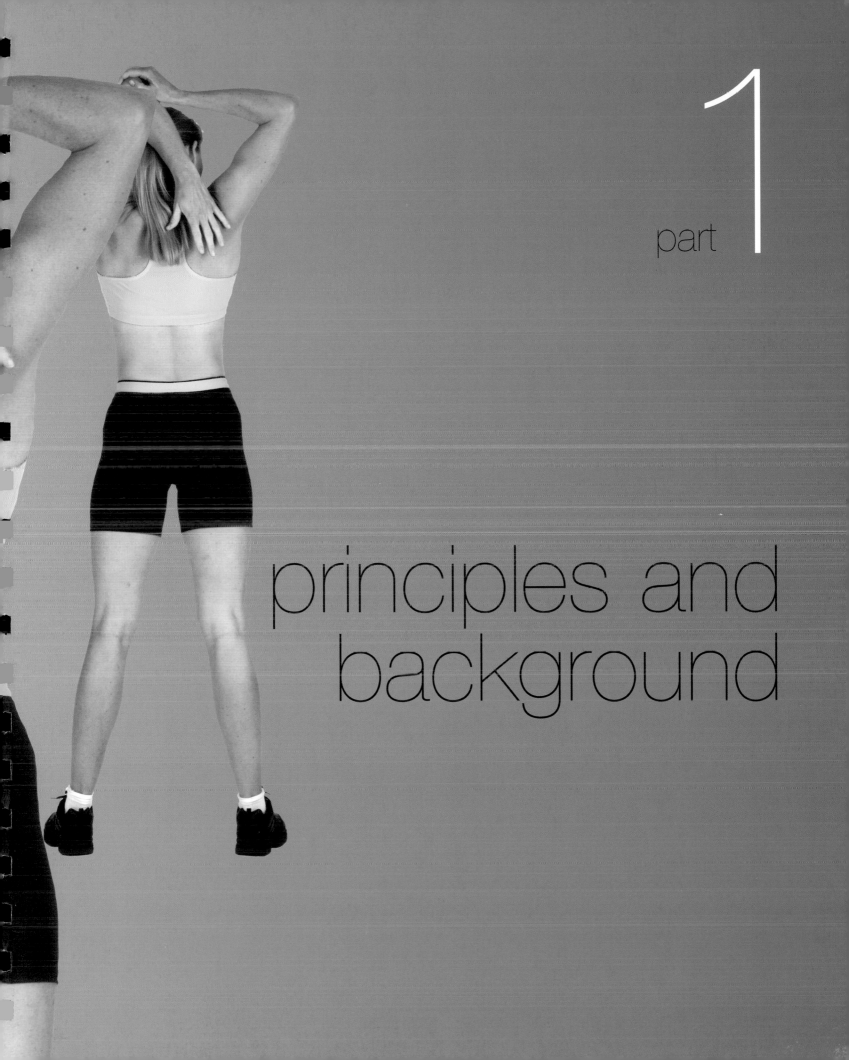

part 1

principles and background

an introduction to the human body

A basic knowledge of anatomy, such as which muscles are where, as well as a general overall understanding of the way the human body functions are vital if we are to form an awareness of the limitations of our own bodies and develop our ability to plan specific exercise programs that are both safe and suitable for training muscles.

the muscular system

Around 40 percent of the body weight of each individual is made up of muscle tissue, with more than five hundred muscles working together in order for the body to function and the limbs to move.

In simple terms, muscles contract (shorten) when certain signals are received from the brain. The muscles are attached to the bones by stretchy tissues called tendons. When the muscles contract, they pull on the tendons, which in turn pull on the bones, causing the limbs to move. For example, in the standing dumbbell curls (pages 58–59), as you raise the weight toward your shoulders, the bicep's role is to pull the forearm toward the shoulder, hence moving the limb.

There are three different types of muscle:
• **smooth muscles** are involuntary, which means that we have no control over their movements and are usually unaware of the work they are doing. Examples of these muscles include the muscles that line the blood vessels, stomach, arteries, digestive tract, and other internal organs. These muscles work continuously, providing a vital role in supporting the body—our bodies would quickly let us down if we had to rely on conscious thought to make these muscles do their jobs.

• **cardiac muscles** are also involuntary. These muscles contract automatically to work the heart, a muscle that has to perform continuously over several decades without ever resting in order to keep us alive.

• **skeletal muscles** are attached to the bones in order to create movement. You should be able to locate the places where the muscles are attached to bones by tendons. See if you can feel the tendons at the back of your knee or in your wrist, for example.

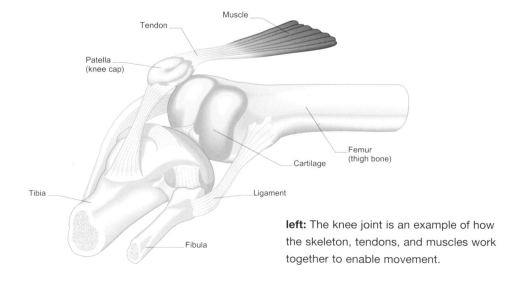

Muscle

Tendon

Patella
(knee cap)

Femur
(thigh bone)

Cartilage

Tibia

Ligament

Fibula

left: The knee joint is an example of how the skeleton, tendons, and muscles work together to enable movement.

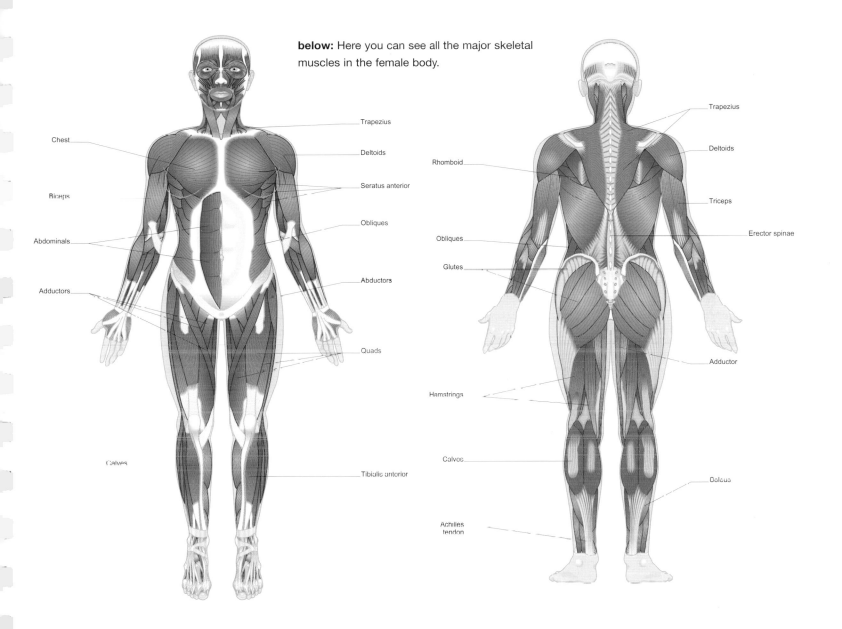

below: Here you can see all the major skeletal muscles in the female body.

Trapezius

Chest

Deltoids

Seratus anterior

Biceps

Obliques

Abdominals

Adductors

Abductors

Quads

Calves

Tibialis anterior

Trapezius

Rhomboid

Deltoids

Triceps

Erector spinae

Obliques

Glutes

Adductor

Hamstrings

Calves

Soleus

Achilles tendon

the skeletal system

As an adult you have only 206 bones in your body, compared to that of an infant with 350. The reason for this difference is that as we grow some of our bones fuse together to form one larger bone. More than half of the 206 bones are found in the hands and feet. Bones are connected to each other by various types of joint, allowing different parts of the body to move in a variety of ways.

Along with providing storage for the red blood cells, the major purpose of the bones is to support and move the body. Some bones, such as the skull or rib cage, are not attached to moveable joints. Their function is to provide protection for delicate internal organs, such as the brain, heart, and lungs.

A tough, smooth, shiny substance called cartilage covers the ends of each bone. The cartilage-coated bone ends are kept apart by a thin film of slippery fluid that works in a similar manner to the oil in a car. This fluid prevents the bones from scratching and knocking against each other as the body moves. Strong stretchy bands called ligaments hold all bones together.

basic strength-training principles

Before plunging into any kind of strength-training program, it is essential that you learn the fundamentals of weight training and training techniques that will help form the basis of your exercise regime. Without learning and understanding this basic knowledge, your progress from beginner to intermediate level will take much longer.

Training without fully understanding what you are doing will only hamper you in achieving the health and fitness goals you have set for yourself and may even cause strain or injury to the body. Building this basic foundation of strength training enables you to effectively establish successful programs that are tailored to your own specific needs and capabilities.

sequence of exercises

As a general rule of thumb, start working the larger muscle groups (such as legs, back, chest, and shoulders) first, using compound movements that employ more than one muscle group to lift the weight. From here, you should progress toward the smaller muscle groups (such as biceps, triceps, calves, and abdominals) that need less energy, focusing more on isolation movements that target a particular muscle.

Training the larger muscle groups at the beginning of your exercise session, when your body is fresh and full of energy, allows for a more efficient and effective workout, rather than struggling at the end of a session to exercise a big muscle group.

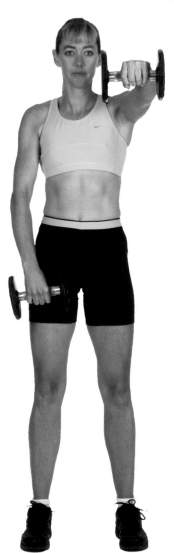
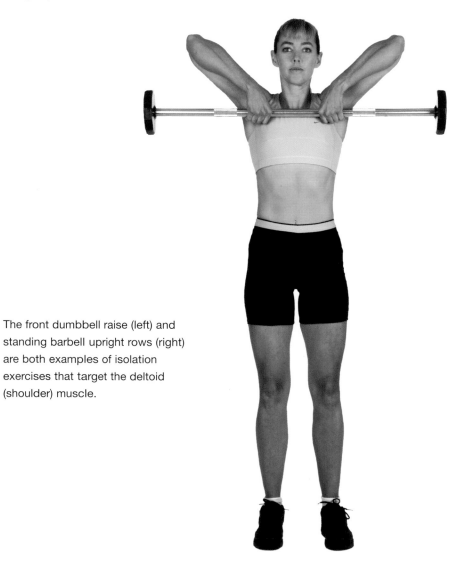

The front dumbbell raise (left) and standing barbell upright rows (right) are both examples of isolation exercises that target the deltoid (shoulder) muscle.

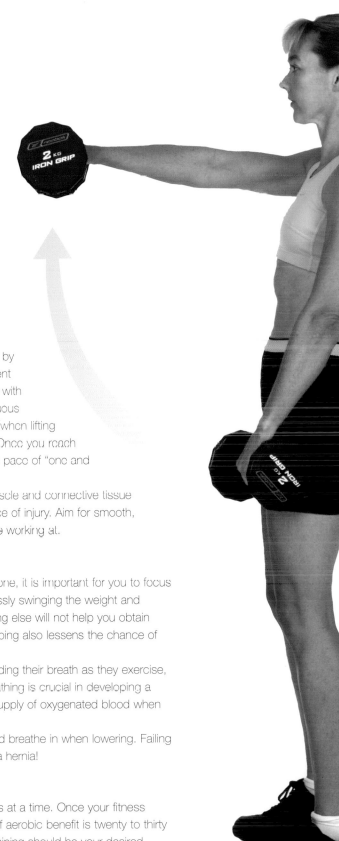

right: Smooth, flowing movement is essential to the safe and effective lifting of weights.

speed

"How fast should I work?" This is a question I'm regularly asked by those starting out. The pace at which you perform any movement makes all the difference between just going through the motion with momentum and actually making the muscle work under continuous tension. An average count of "one and two and three and . . ." when lifting and lowering weights is a good training pace for the beginner. Once you reach intermediate level and have mastered the beginner exercises, a pace of "one and two and . . ." on lifting and lowering the weight is sufficient.

Performing fast, jerky, uneven movements will place the muscle and connective tissue under unnecessary stress and considerably increase the chance of injury. Aim for smooth, flowing, continuous movement, whatever level or speed you are working at.

concentration and breathing

When training, whether you are lifting a light weight or a heavy one, it is important for you to focus your concentration on the muscle that you are working. Mindlessly swinging the weight and simply going through the motions while thinking about something else will not help you obtain your strength-training goals. Focusing totally on what you are doing also lessens the chance of accidental injury or muscle strain.

On countless occasions I have seen people in the gym holding their breath as they exercise, as if they were swimming underwater. Correct, continuous breathing is crucial in developing a good technique, as your muscles and brain need a constant supply of oxygenated blood when lifting weights.

As a general guide, breathe out when raising the weight and breathe in when lowering. Failing to breathe correctly can lead to broken blood vessels or even a hernia!

training duration

As a novice trainer you may only be able to train for ten minutes at a time. Once your fitness increases the minimum length of time to exercise for any sort of aerobic benefit is twenty to thirty minutes. Combined with strength training, around an hour of training should be your desired exercise time.

However, the duration will depend on your level of ability—whether you are a complete novice or an intermediate—how quickly you learn the exercises and the time that you have available to train in. As I say to my clients, ten minutes is better than no minutes!

sets and repetitions

When you think about strength training, think about sets and reps (repetitions). The latter is the key to the former. A set means doing one exercise continuously with a certain number of successive repetitions performed without resting. Reps are the number of times you repeat the move in each set. For example if you are told to do 3 sets of 12 repetitions (3 x 12 reps) of standing dumbbell curls, you would curl the weight 12 times continuously, counting this as one full set. Then you'd rest for a moment and stretch the bicep muscle (see section on stretching) before completing the next set of 12 reps, and so on, until you have completed the full 3 sets of 12 reps.

Sets and reps give structure to your strength-training routine, allowing you to gauge how hard your body is working (by the last couple of reps it should be a real challenge to keep lifting the weight) and imposing the discipline you need to keep training the muscle. If you want to plan your routine of sets and repetitions you can use a table like this one.

	No. of repetitions	Name of exercise
Set 1		
Set 2		
Set 3		

range of movement

The amount of weight you can lift will depend on how naturally strong you are and how long you have been training. It is important that sufficient weight is used for you to feel the muscle working, but not so much that you struggle with the movement and cause injury to yourself. As a rule, heavy weights are used for strength, power, and more advanced strength training; medium–heavy weights for building muscle; and light–medium weights for endurance and toning.

Using the full range of movement of the muscles as you carry each exercise through from start to finish strengthens and stretches the muscles; you are working to improve both muscle strength and tone and joint flexibility. Every exercise should be taken through the complete range of joint movement in a slow, controlled manner. Lifting the weight only halfway or having to swing or jerk it up and down means that the weight is too heavy for you at this stage. There is no point in using the incorrect form or overly heavy weights over a full range of movement—you are only cheating yourself out of gaining the best results possible from your workout. You will develop much more quickly if you perform an exercise correctly, using lighter weights that are more suited to your current level of ability.

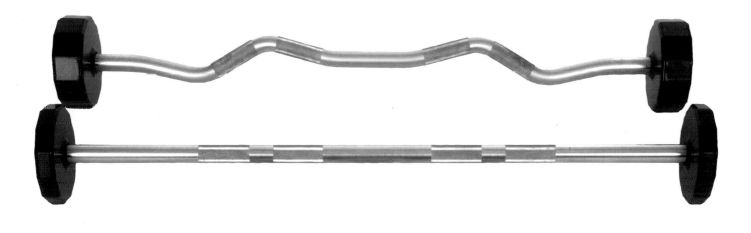

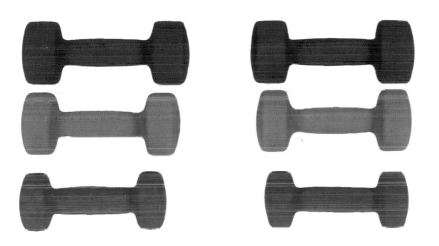

left: A full range of free weights should be available to any trainer, but it is important that you choose the right weight for your strength and ability. Here you can see (from the top) the EZ bar, barbell, and a variety of dumbbells.

overload

Simply put, this means exercising the muscle slightly above the level at which it feels absolutely comfortable. You are "overloading" the muscle and the effect of this is to make the muscle work harder and ultimately become stronger and increase the lean muscle mass. Challenge your muscles in this way every time or every second time you work out and it will lead to constant progress in your training. Some overload techniques are outlined in the section on basic training techniques.

the plateau

The "plateau" is the imaginary wall that you hit when you begin to lose faith in your training—you may even stop exercising when results seem to come to a grinding halt. When the body and mind are not being challenged by your training routine, then you seriously need to consider varying and adjusting your exercise sessions. This may be a good time to find a strength instructor to assess how you have been training and what can be done to improve your routine, before you hit reversibility.

reversibility

This is the stage after the plateau and it occurs if you stop working out completely. If you don't train often enough or with sufficient intensity to overload the muscle each time, the benefits of exercising are quickly lost. This is why it's important to train regularly—if only to maintain what you have already achieved through your workouts so far.

basic training techniques

Here are a few of the most commonly used basic training techniques.

blitzing

This technique involves bombarding a specific muscle or muscles with a variety of different exercises that work the muscle(s) in different ways.

pyramid sets

This is a high intensity training technique whereby you deliberately overload the muscle, increasing the weight after each set and using reasonably low repetitions (6–10 reps) until the muscle becomes totally fatigued. Muscles adapt very quickly to sets, reps, and resistance as well as to regular routines. Progressively overloading the muscle will give dramatic results.

compound training (super sets, tri sets, giant sets)

Here you use a group of training techniques that combines exercises for the same muscle and/or opposite muscles such as biceps/triceps or back/chest. Don't rest between these exercises.

super sets

This method works one muscle group or opposite muscle groups such as back/chest. An example of working opposite muscle groups would be leg extensions followed by machine lying leg curls. An example of working the same muscle group would be incline dumbbell press followed by machine pec deck.

tri sets

This technique works the same body part. An example of this would be using a series of exercises such as flat bench dumbbell presses, incline dumbbell presses, and machine pec deck to work the chest.

giant sets

These are super sets with more than two exercises for the same body part with no rest in between. For example: leg press, leg extensions, Swiss-ball squats, and then lunges.

preexhaustion

This technique works to specifically isolate any given muscle before overloading it with a compound movement that works more than one muscle group. This is a great technique for preventing secondary muscles from coming into play before working the main muscle you are trying to target. An example of this would be dumbbell side raises followed by dumbbell presses.

circuit training

below: A combination of exercises should train the upper, middle, and lower body on lying, standing, and seated machines. To start you off, you can try the following combination:

Circuit training takes you quickly through a series of exercises on a variety of fixed-weight machines. Do one set of exercise on a machine and then move on to the next with no rest in between. This technique gets the heart pumping and the whole body working hard and is a great way to improve overall fitness and strength as well as introduce weight training to the novice strength trainer. It is also a good technique to use when your time is limited.

START	bike	back	thighs	abdominals
bike	chest	hamstrings	calves	bike
shoulders	abdominals	arms	bike	FINISH

guidelines for strength training

The following are some basic guidelines that you should adhere to during any strength-training routine.

1 Always set aside five to ten minutes at the beginning and the end for warming up and cooling down your muscles. The amount of time should be increased in cold weather.

2 Pay attention to the correct form of the exercise and the safe use of all equipment. Strain and injury can happen very quickly and without warning and can set you back weeks, if not months, depending on the type of injury.

3 Always maintain a slight bend in your elbows and knees when training, as this takes the tension off the ligaments and joints, reducing the risk of stress and strain to these areas. Always make sure that you perform a full range of movement from the start to the finish of each exercise.

4 Avoid lifting too much weight too soon — this is yet another way of causing yourself injury. Also make sure you breathe correctly while training (see page 13).

5 Spread your workouts evenly throughout the week rather than cramming everything into one session. Trying to do everything at once and too intensely can cause you to burn out and lose enthusiasm. Over-training can also lead to a depleted immune system, hampering results and leading to illness. Put simply, you will wear yourself out.

6 Always stretch before and between exercises and at the end of your training session to relieve muscle soreness and cramping and to increase the flexibility of the muscles.

7 Make sure you drink enough water before, during, and after training to avoid dehydration and ensure that your body can function properly, as the body uses far more fluid when exercising. As you sweat you lose water, which needs to be replaced quickly. A minimum of two liters a day is needed, more in hotter climates or when training more intensely.

8 Allow enough time between training sessions for your body to rest properly, so that it is fresh for the next workout. Larger muscle groups may need three to four days of rest while smaller muscles need only two to three days. Training every day will ultimately work against your general fitness levels and can cause your muscles to feel constantly tired and reluctant to work.

9 If you have any medical problems, are pregnant, taking medication, or have prior injuries or any health concerns at all, please consult your doctor or qualified strength instructor before starting any strength-training or exercise program.

10 What you do outside of your training sessions is just as important as the training itself. Make sure that you eat healthily, minimize your alcohol intake, and reduce the amount of saturated fat in your diet. If you smoke, try to gradually cut the number of cigarettes you smoke. Seek sound nutritional advice from a qualified instructor or nutritionist if you are unsure of your needs or have any doubts about how to structure a healthy, balanced diet.

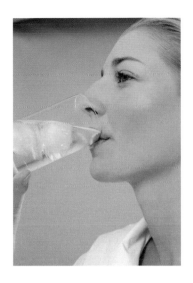

above: Regular sips of water are crucial to safe and comfortable strength training, keeping the body hydrated while exercising. It is also a good idea to drink water at regular intervals throughout the day as part of your routine.

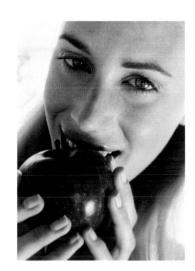

above: Healthy eating is just as important as regular visits to the gym for both your general health and strength training.

free weights vs. machines

One of the most commonly asked questions in strength training is "Should I use free weights or machines?" The answer is: *both*.

You'll find that opinions vary on this subject, with some people swearing by free weights while others insist that machines are the only way to go. Both have a great deal to offer, though you should also take into account whether you are an absolute beginner or closer to the intermediate level. For beginners, machines have the advantage of requiring little skill or coordination. They support your body in a fixed position and guide you through the movement from start to finish. Machines also help isolate muscle groups and almost guarantee correct training technique.

Free weights, on the other hand, require a certain degree of coordination and stability, but the movement is able to be far more natural, mimicking real-life movement more accurately. Free weights incorporate other muscle groups into a movement as well as the muscle that you are specifically training. Several muscles are required to shift, balance, and steady the body as you raise and lower a free weight.

As a novice it is very important that you learn the necessary skills to handle free weights correctly, developing the proper technique and correct posture so that you don't injure yourself. This does not mean that you should omit free weights as you start to train; just make sure you have received proper guidance from a qualified strength instructor.

A strength trainer needs to be versatile and willing to utilize all the various pieces of equipment and training opportunities that the gym has to offer. One regular complaint about strength training is that it can become monotonous and boring. This often has to do with the unadventurous approach the trainer brings to the gym: if you repeatedly use the same fixed or free weights in the same order and the same number of repetitions in every session, you are quickly going to become bored. Vary the order of your routine and experiment with your weights—don't be frightened of them. Here are a few of the pros and cons of free weights and machines to consider.

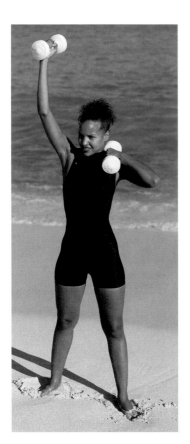

above: Free weights have the advantage of being portable, so you can use them anywhere to maintain and enjoy your strength-training routine.

free weights

advantages
- Allow a wide variety of exercises to be performed
- Teach coordination, since the exercise is not predetermined as with machines
- Are inexpensive, portable, versatile
- Are suitable for all shapes and sizes
- Create a more natural movement than similar moves performed on machines

disadvantages
- Require more supervision (particularly for the novice), as the risk of injury is greater
- May require another person to help you with your training
- Exclude certain exercises, such as leg press and leg extensions
- Require lower back support or strong back and abdominal muscles for certain exercises such as squats or any standing overhead movement
- Demand that you remember more about how to perform each exercise safely and correctly
- Can be intimidating to novice trainers, especially women

machines

advantages

- Require less supervision
- Provide support of the lower back with the backrest
- Demand less knowledge about how to do each movement safely and correctly
- Are user friendly, relatively more comfortable, and can be less intimidating to beginners and women
- Provide less risk of strain or injury
- Allow you to focus on a major muscle group, rather than including other, smaller muscle groups that help you lift the weight from start to finish
- Are good for rehabilitation of injuries, since you are in a fixed position

disadvantages

- Are expensive to buy and repair
- Can be large and impractical to have at home
- Are often intended for only one exercise
- Are usually designed for the average size person, so finding a piece of equipment that feels comfortable can be a problem
- Allow for less improvement in coordination and stability, since muscles other than the large (stabilizer) muscle groups are not usually activated

below: The simple push-up uses your own body weight to strength train. You don't need either fixed or free weights for this exercise.

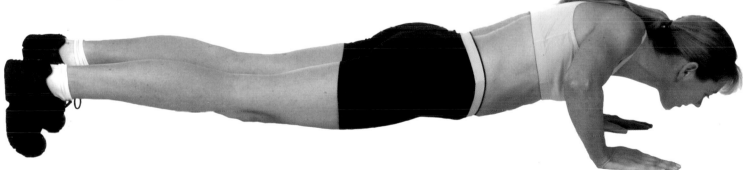

The foundation of your training is to create a balanced, well-shaped, and toned physique. Free weights and machines are both fantastic, but don't overlook the cheapest and most versatile piece of equipment you could ever use as resistance—your own body! From crunches to push-ups, indoors or outdoors, your workout is waiting for you.

common strength-training myths

fact vs. fiction

There are possibly more myths and misconceptions surrounding strength training than any other physical activity. This is due largely to a combination of ignorance and fear. Many people have never stepped into a gym because they are intimidated by the machines and afraid of making fools of themselves. Or perhaps they're scared of developing huge muscles, which they believe will immediately turn to fat when they stop lifting. None of these fears are justified. Below I've outlined some of the major strength-training misconceptions—and then blasted them out of the water with the real exercise facts.

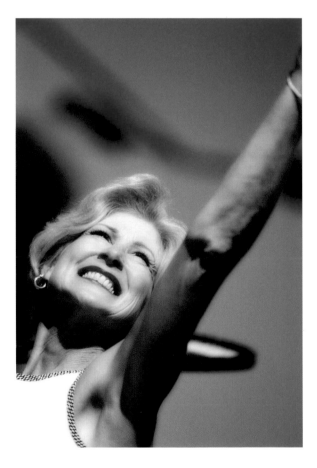

above: Strength training is an important part of an older woman's fitness regime. It guards against osteoporosis and improves coordination, helping her enjoy a variety of sports.

Fiction: Strength training is no help with weight loss.

Fact: Some people think that because strength training is not a high-level aerobic workout, it doesn't help you lose weight. But strength training should be integrated into any exercise routine. Aerobic training and strength training together provide the perfect balance of exercise to improve your fitness and give you a leaner body.

Dieting alone doesn't work. The scales may tell you you're losing weight, but this weight loss is partly due to dwindling muscle and reduced water content in the body. Losing your muscle tissue has a direct impact on your ability to lose weight, as it causes your body's metabolism to slow down. This means that when you come off the diet and start eating normally, your body will put on weight more easily than if you had never dieted at all.

But with strength training, you can maintain or increase lean muscle, which in turn will maintain or increase your metabolism—improving your ability to burn off fat. Your muscles are the key to burning extra calories when active and at rest. The more lean muscle mass you have, the more efficient your body will be.

Fiction: Strength training will make a woman look like the Incredible Hulk!

Fact: Virtually every woman faced with the prospect of strength training has said, "I don't want to develop bulging muscles." But the truth is that most women aren't capable of building huge muscles, even if they try. Women don't have the genetic capacity to build muscular size the way men do, nor do we have the high levels of the muscle-building hormone testosterone.

Most women will have to work reasonably hard to obtain a slight increase in lean muscle, let alone developing bulk. But strength training will result in a leaner and more toned physique. Genetics play a part, of course, and some women will be able to tone their muscles more quickly than others. But by and large, women don't have to worry about rippling muscles getting in the way of their femininity.

Fiction: Strength training is dangerous for seniors.

Fact: It's never too late to start strength training; it improves coordination and strengthens bones, which is an important consideration, since osteoporosis is a real danger—particularly for women—as you get older. Through regular physical activity the muscles remain strong and well toned, the body maintains its flexibility, and the chances of illness and injury are greatly reduced.

Fiction: Abdominal exercises will remove fat from around your stomach and make it flat.

Fact: Fat and muscle are two completely different tissue types. The idea of turning fat into muscle is unrealistic. Abdominal exercises strengthen and tone your stomach muscles, but if there's any excess fat lying on top of your muscles, no one is going to be able to admire your six-pack. The only answer is to combine abdominal exercises with the loss of unwanted fat through aerobic training. So don't devote your entire exercise routine to crunching, because spot reduction doesn't work.

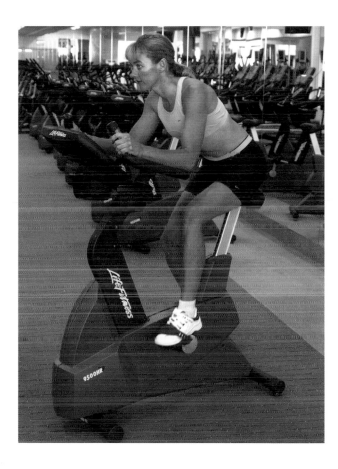

left: Aerobic training is an essential partner to strength training if you want to lose unwanted fat.

Fiction: Your muscles will turn to fat if you stop strength training.

Fact: This is my all-time favorite myth. Muscle cannot turn into fat—but it *can* be replaced by it if you stop exercising and start overeating. When you stop strength training, inevitably your muscles will lose their tone and size, and if you continue to take in calories you no longer need, you are obviously going to gain fat. If you do stop training completely, for any reason, make sure you lower your calorie consumption, particularly because you will not be burning calories as efficiently as when you were exercising regularly. Always adjust your eating habits according to the amount of exercise you do.

Fiction: If you are thin you don't need to exercise.

Fact: Regardless of your body shape and size, you need to exercise. A slender body is no indication at all of your fitness level—you may simply be genetically predisposed to be thin. You could also be genetically predisposed to some unseen vulnerability, such as heart disease, so it is crucial for you to exercise your body and that most important muscle, the heart. A slight frame is also far more vulnerable to bone fractures—all the more reason to train to strengthen your bones and build your muscles up.

benefits of strength training

Many women tend to rely mainly on aerobic training and fad dieting to control their body weight, but if you want to see any change in your body shape, the real significance of strength training for women cannot be underestimated. It is now recognized to be an integral part of any fitness regime, and, along with activities that focus on weight control and flexibility, strength training ensures a well-balanced, injury-free lifestyle, whatever your age. From adolescents right through to octogenarians, strength training has proven benefits for all age groups. Here are just a few of the many benefits of strength training.

❶ Increases metabolic rate. Strength training increases the body's metabolism, causing you to burn more calories both while exercising and at rest.

❷ Increases and restores bone density. Inactivity and aging lead to a decrease in bone density and cause brittle bones. Strength training is capable of drastically increasing your bone density and thereby preventing osteoporosis.

❸ Increases lean muscle mass and muscle strength, power, and aerobic endurance. Everyone can benefit from being stronger—daily activity becomes easier, sex drive may increase, and we find ourselves able to enjoy our lives better and be more physically active.

❹ Strengthens muscles and joints. This can prevent a wide variety of injuries.

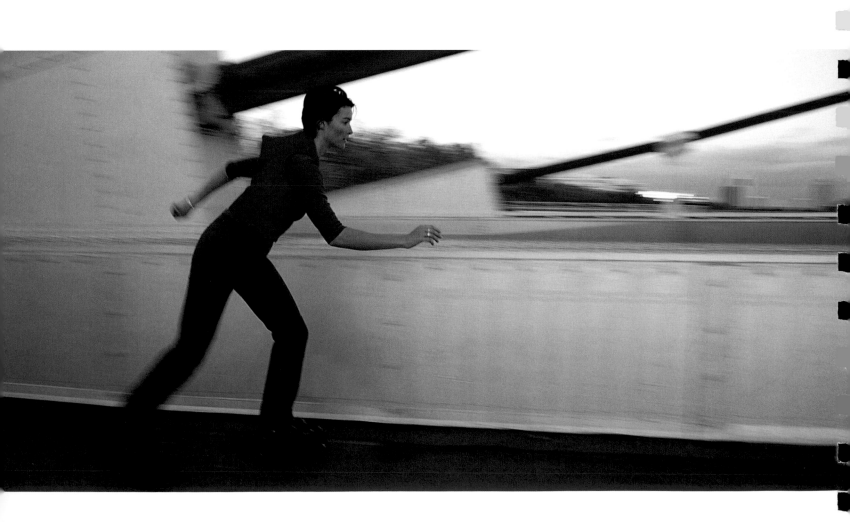

❺ Decreases risk of diseases. Regular strength training has a diverse range of health benefits, including decreasing cholesterol and lowering your blood pressure, reducing stress, and improving sleep patterns. It can also help with glucose tolerance, insulin sensitivity, and coronary disease.

❻ Aids rehabilitation and recovery. Muscles need to go through rehab programs following injury. Strength training is seen as one of the best ways to heal an injury, as it strengthens the surrounding muscles and speeds up the healing process.

❼ Increases sports performance. A strength program can dramatically improve your performance and technique in other physical activities.

❽ Encourages an elegant aging process. Physical activity keeps us feeling young and lively. Strong, healthy seniors have good coordination, balance, and flexibility and consequently suffer from fewer accidents. If they do fall, their bodies are more resilient, they are less likely to be injured, and they are able to heal more quickly if they do sustain any injury.

❾ Improves our feeling of overall well-being. There is nothing more fulfilling than the invigorated feeling after a satisfying workout. Stronger muscles and joints can have a dramatic impact on posture, and leaner, toned muscles tend to improve an individual's self-esteem, confidence, and feeling of well-being.

❿ Strength training can be adapted to all levels of fitness. Regardless of whether you are a novice or an intermediate, strength training can be adjusted to suit your particular needs.

left: Strength training benefits all other sports you take part in, improving performance and technique.

right: Lifting weights infuses your body with a sense of well-being and encourages a positive mental outlook.

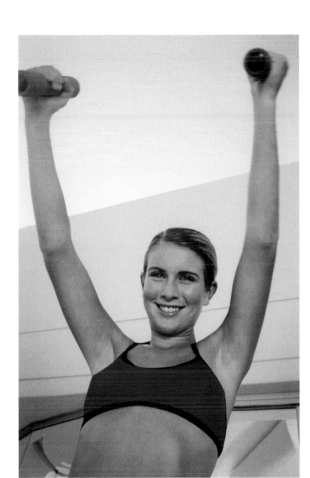

your body type

Strength training is not something you should do mindlessly, repeating a set of specific exercises. You need to develop an understanding of your body and how it works; this will greatly affect your training and your ability to achieve the goals you have set for yourself.

Body typing, also called somatotyping, was developed by the psychologist Dr. William H. Sheldon in the 1940s to classify people according to the shape of their body. Not everyone responds to training in exactly the same way, so what works for one person may not work so well for someone else. Once you are familiar with your body type and its particular needs, you will be able to tailor your training and goals.

the three basic body types

endomorph

Endomorphs are round in shape with a softer physical appearance. Often pear shaped with a round head, they carry a high percentage of body fat, usually around the lower body—mainly on the hips and stomach.

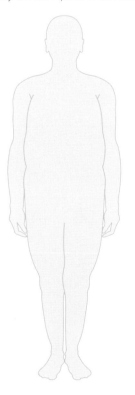

mesomorph

Mesomorphs are usually V-shaped, with narrow hips and broad shoulders. They may be quite muscular and strong. People with this body type tend to have normal- to below-average body fat levels.

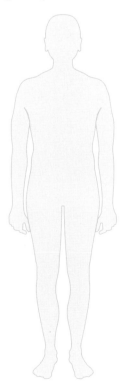

ectomorph

Ectomorphs are lean and long in appearance. They are often characterized by their short trunk and long limbs, with narrow shoulders, hips, chest, and abdomen. Ectomorphs have little or no fat or muscle.

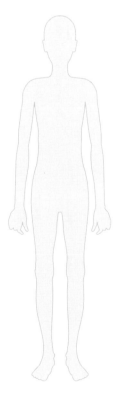

It is quite common to have characteristics of more than one body type. For example, you might be an endo-meso or meso-ecto.

Your body type is determined by genetics and no amount of strength training can alter what you were born with. If you happen to be an endomorph, all the training in the world will not make you an ectomorph. But you can improve on what you've been given. With the right kind of training you can lose your excess body fat and tone your muscles, creating a leaner body shape.

training your body type

How do you train best to suit your body type? Here are some general rules:

• Because of their body shape, endomorphs tend to have a higher percentage of body fat and usually have to work harder to lose it. If you do have this body type, you need to be vigilant when strength training, since added muscle mass can make your physique look bulky and large rather than slimmer and leaner. Endomorphs are usually best suited to swimming, very light, high-repetition weight training, walking, and aerobic classes.

• Mesomorphs, on the other hand, because of their naturally muscular, athletic physique, lose body fat quickly and gain muscular size easily. Muscular mesomorphs are ideal for any type of strength or power sport, such as weight training, power lifting, sprinting, boxing, wrestling, and even martial arts.

• Lanky ectomorphs tend to make great long-distance runners, bikers, power walkers, and aerobic exercisers. Ectomorphs usually have a faster metabolism and tend to lose body fat easily, but, because of their long slender limbs, they have to work harder to achieve any type of muscular definition.

• Always remember to work with your body type, not against it. Below are some pretraining questions to consider; these will encourage you to focus on what you can achieve. Before you set foot in the gym, take a piece of paper and write down the answers to these questions.

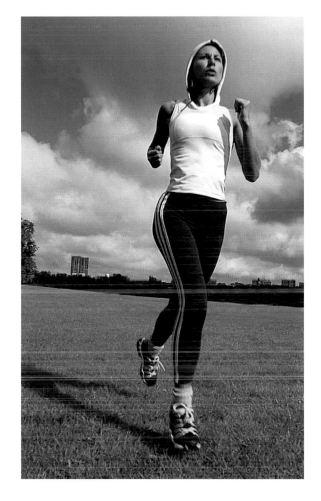

right: Power sports such as sprinting suit mesomorphs.

❶ "What goal do I ultimately wish to achieve in my strength-training routine?"

❷ "Can I clearly define my short-, mid-, and long-term goals?"

❸ "Are the exercises that I'm doing gradually altering the shape of my body in line with these goals?"

❹ "Am I happy with how my body is changing? If not, what steps am I going to take to change this feeling?"

❺ "Do I fully understand what body type I am, since it's important to know how my body will react to certain sports and exercises?"

Put this piece of paper in a prominent place—such as on the refrigerator door—where you know you will see it every day. It will help sustain your motivation and ensure that you remember what you are meant to be doing and why. Naturally, your answers will change as you progress, so it's crucial that they are updated from time to time.

the importance of aerobic and anaerobic training

Achieving your ultimate goal isn't just about hitting the weights day in, day out. Strength training shouldn't—and can't—work in isolation. You also need to include a program of aerobic and anaerobic exercises in your routine to complement your work in the gym.

the benefit of aerobic training

"Aerobic exercise"—or "cardiovascular fitness" or "cardio," as it's frequently referred to—is central to any weight-management system. Essentially, aerobic training is any form of continuous exercise that uses the large muscles in your body and relies on oxygen to supply the body's energy.

When exercising aerobically, the heart and lungs work harder, which has the effect of improving their function and therefore decreasing the risk of heart disease. The body's need for oxygen increases with the intensity of exercise—regular exercise improves your body's ability to move higher levels of oxygenated blood through the heart and lungs.

The key benefit of aerobic training comes when your body exploits its own energy sources (stored carbohydrates and fats) more efficiently in the presence of oxygen-fueled energy. Put simply, when you work your body aerobically it starts to burn up stored fat in order to supply the muscles with an instant source of energy. Working aerobically also increases your long-term metabolic rate so that you burn calories more efficiently and at a higher rate even when resting, thus helping you to keep your weight under control.

Besides the countless physical benefits that come with aerobic training, there are also psychological effects that contribute to your overall state of well-being. Activity encourages the body to release endorphins, the body's "feel good hormones"—so exercise can actually make you feel happy, and feeling good is surprisingly compulsive! Also, as you start to see the results of your hard work, your confidence levels will increase, your mind will become clearer, and you will notice improvement in your concentration.

In addition, vigorous exercise provides you with the perfect way of working off any stress or frustration in a positive way. And for those who have trouble sleeping, exercise can help regulate your sleep patterns so that you wake feeling rested and refreshed.

right: Feeling good is a surprising and positive side effect of strength training. You'll have more energy for other forms of exercise, too.

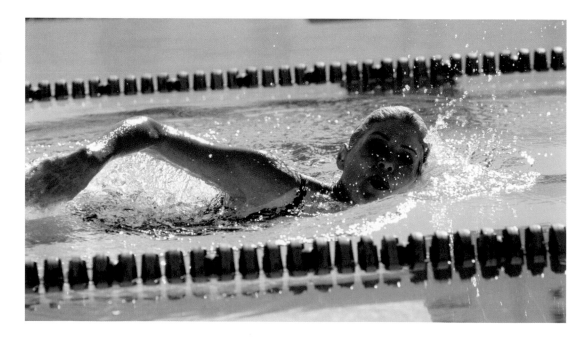

the benefit of anaerobic training

Anaerobic training is the opposite of exercising aerobically, as you produce energy without using extra oxygen. It is very easy to switch from aerobic to anaerobic training—for example, by shifting from jogging to sprinting. Increasing the intensity of aerobic training moves you to a point where your cardiorespiratory system cannot supply enough oxygen to sustain your training aerobically, so the body quickly changes to an anaerobic system.

The form of intense, focused exercise found in strength training teaches your body to withstand the onset of fatigue and push past the pain barrier, allowing it to develop the ability to train harder and longer.

In anaerobic training your body's energy source is glycogen (carbohydrate that has been broken down as fuel for the body's cells, such as muscle glycogen). But the source of glycogen rapidly starts to deplete, so the body becomes more reliant on using stored fat as its main source of energy production. Since training anaerobically is more intense than aerobic exercise, far more calories are burned.

You will be able to maintain high-intensity, anaerobic exercise for only short bursts of time before you need to stop and catch your breath. However, by combining both aerobic and anaerobic training, you can achieve lean muscle mass and increased metabolism.

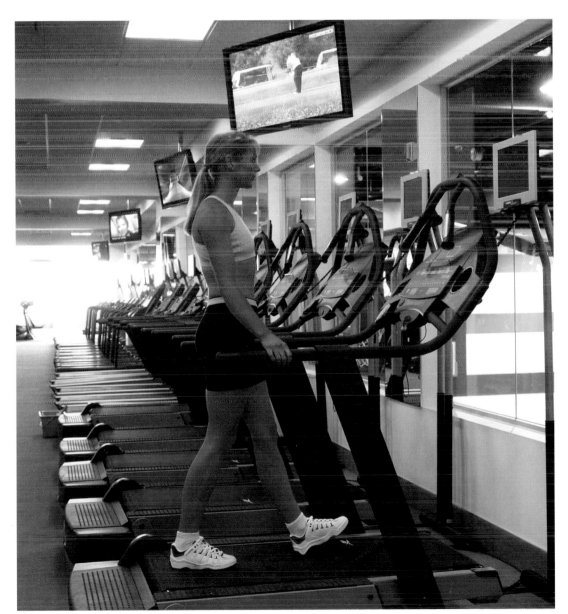

left: The treadmill can provide you with crucial anaerobic exercise—just shift from jogging to sprinting.

the importance of stretching

Regular stretching of the muscles before you start, between exercises, and at the end of your session is an essential part of training. But stretching is also an important part of daily life. Lack of exercise, the aging process, and neglecting to stretch regularly causes your muscles to gradually lose their elasticity and flexibility. This means that any urgent and sudden movement of the body might demand a level of strength and flexibility that you just don't have, resulting in injury or damage to the muscle tissue.

However, before you begin stretching, you also need to be aware of the dangers of muscles becoming too flexible. The overflexibility of a muscle can occur when it is stretched beyond its maximum length. This can lead to your joints becoming hypermobile, losing their stability as they are extended beyond their own limitations. Ligaments and tendons are put under unnecessary stress and the overflexible muscles become less effective at protecting your joints, which can lead to injuries. So, be wary of excessive flexibility. A ligament stretched 6 percent beyond its normal length will eventually tear.

benefits of stretching

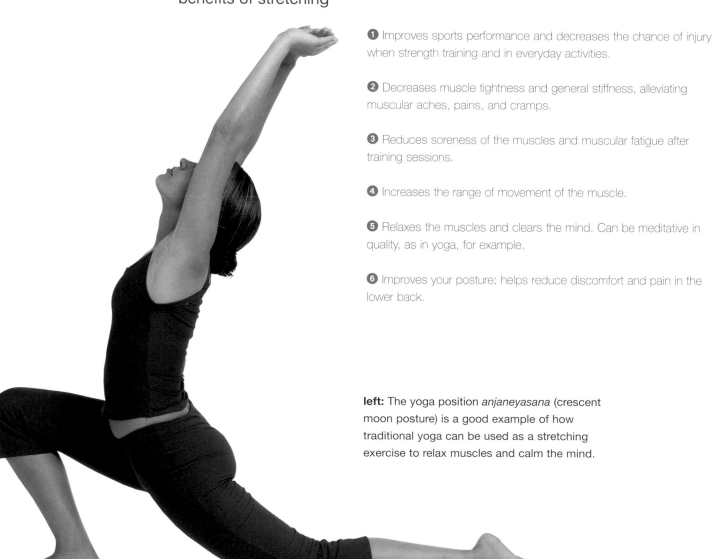

❶ Improves sports performance and decreases the chance of injury when strength training and in everyday activities.

❷ Decreases muscle tightness and general stiffness, alleviating muscular aches, pains, and cramps.

❸ Reduces soreness of the muscles and muscular fatigue after training sessions.

❹ Increases the range of movement of the muscle.

❺ Relaxes the muscles and clears the mind. Can be meditative in quality, as in yoga, for example.

❻ Improves your posture; helps reduce discomfort and pain in the lower back.

left: The yoga position *anjaneyasana* (crescent moon posture) is a good example of how traditional yoga can be used as a stretching exercise to relax muscles and calm the mind.

types of stretches

There are seven main types of stretches:

ballistic stretching

This consists of stretching the muscle to the limit of its normal range of motion, then overstretching it by bouncing the stretched muscle. It uses the stretched muscle as a springboard to stretch the muscle even further. Ballistic stretching does not allow the muscles to adjust to or relax into the stretched position. This type of stretching is *not* recommended as it can lead to injury.

dynamic stretching

Unlike ballistic stretching, dynamic stretching consists of controlled leg and arm swings that gently take the muscles to the limit of their range of movement. There are no bouncing or jerky movements here. This type of stretching improves dynamic flexibility and is useful as part of your warm-up for active or aerobic workouts (such as dancing or martial arts). Examples of this sort of stretch would be slow, controlled leg swings, arm swings, or torso twists.

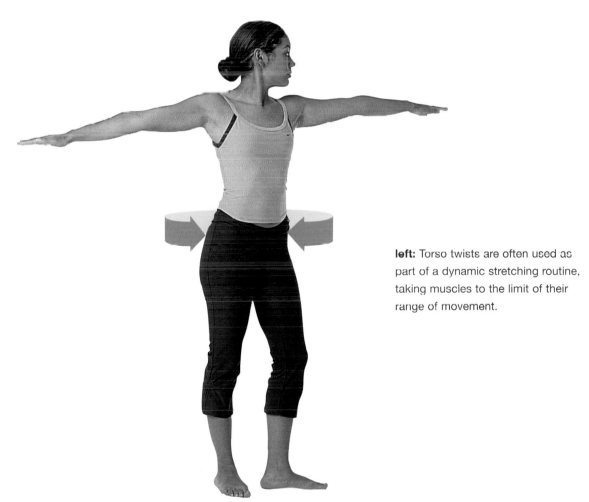

left: Torso twists are often used as part of a dynamic stretching routine, taking muscles to the limit of their range of movement.

active stretching

Active stretching is also referred to as "static-active" stretching, "dynamic," or "range of movement" stretching and involves assuming a particular stretch position and then holding it, using only the strength of the muscle being stretched. For example, extend your leg up in front of you and then hold it there without assistance (using only the leg muscles themselves). This type of stretching increases flexibility and strengthens your muscles. However, it can be difficult to sustain for more than ten seconds and rarely needs to be held longer than fifteen seconds. Many yoga movements are active stretches.

passive (or relaxed) stretching

Passive stretching is also referred to as "relaxed" stretching or "static-passive" stretching. It involves gradually stretching (without bouncing) the muscle to a comfortable point and holding for twenty to thirty seconds—it can be done alone or with the assistance of a partner or apparatus. This type of stretching is useful in relieving spasms in muscles that are healing after an injury and is also a good way to cool down after a workout, as it helps reduce postworkout muscle fatigue and soreness. I would recommend passive stretching to beginners and intermediates alike. It is safe and effective and stretches the muscle and connective tissue in a controlled manner.

static stretching

You will find that the terms "passive stretching" and "static stretching" are used interchangeably. However, there is a subtle difference between the two:

Static stretching involves holding a position—you stretch to the furthest point comfortable and then hold the stretch.

Passive stretching involves assuming a position and then relaxing into a stretch using gravity, a training partner, or a piece of equipment.

isometric stretching

Isometric stretching is similar to static stretching in that it doesn't use motion. This form of stretching involves the resistance of other muscle groups through isometric contractions (tensing) of the stretched muscles. For example, an isometric calf stretch, which uses a wall to provide resistance, is known as the "push-the-wall" calf stretch. (Since children and adolescents are usually naturally flexible, they have no need to perform this type of stretch; their bones are still growing, so there is a chance they could damage connective tissue and tendons.)

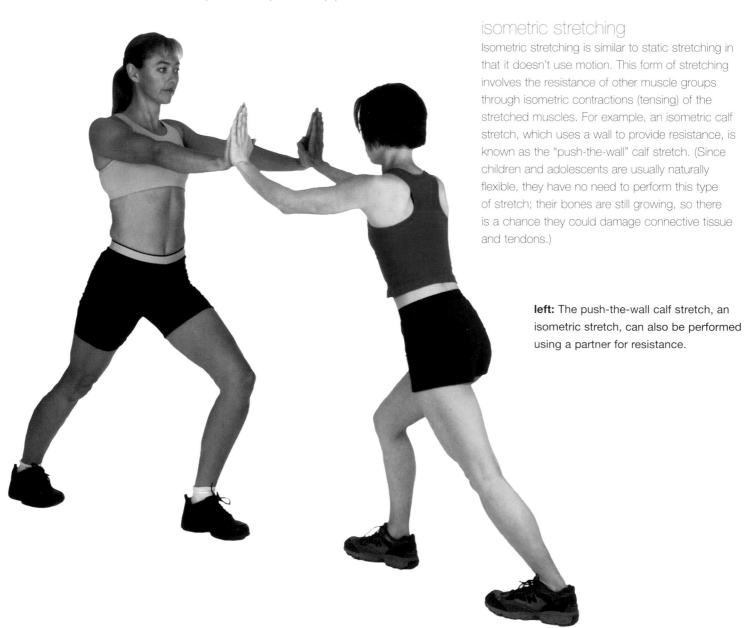

left: The push-the-wall calf stretch, an isometric stretch, can also be performed using a partner for resistance.

PNF stretching

Proprioceptive neuromuscular facilitation (PNF) stretching is presently the quickest and most practical way of stretching, and it is known to increase static-passive flexibility. A PNF stretch involves a static stretch directly followed by an isometric contraction of the muscle against a fixed resistance such as a training partner. The muscle is then stretched even further, statically, before the identical stretch is repeated. PNF stretching is ideal for both beginners and intermediates; it is best practiced under the guidance of a qualified instructor.

when should you stretch?

Every day! At your desk, while watching TV, or even when standing in the kitchen making a cup of coffee—anytime you feel stiff, or whenever your muscles cramp, and, of course, as part of your strength-training program. Five or ten minutes a day is all that is required to maintain your flexibility.

You should stretch as part of your warm up routine and between sets of exercises, because strength training, by causing the muscles to tighten and shorten, actually reduces flexibility. Stretching in the cool-down phase of your training session also helps to relax the muscle and ease any soreness or cramping associated with strength training.

guidelines for stretching

The following are basic guidelines for undertaking any form of flexibility training routine.

1 Avoid holding your breath when stretching; make sure your breathing is slow and constant.

2 Stretch to the point where it's comfortable. Never push yourself beyond your own limit.

3 Only stretch muscles that are already warm. Never try to stretch a cold muscle—this can lead to strain and injury. In very cold weather or climates make sure that you wear sufficient clothing to keep your muscles warm while stretching.

4 Mentally focus on the muscle that is being stretched, concentrating on relaxing it.

5 Avoid bouncy, jerky movements.

6 Pregnant women should stretch only under supervision. During pregnancy a hormone called relaxin is released to aid childbirth. It causes the tendons and ligaments to soften, making the body more flexible than usual. Women can suffer serious injuries if they overstretch while this hormone is present in the body.

7 If you need to stop regular stretching because of an injury, it is essential that you seek qualified advice before starting again.

8 Hold each stretch for twenty to thirty seconds.

9 Stretch every day to maintain flexibility. An increase in flexibility can be noticed in as little as a couple of weeks when stretching is practiced regularly, and flexibility can be quickly lost if it is not done regularly.

warming up and cooling down

Warming up and cooling down should form an integral part of any exercise program. A well-orchestrated warm-up and cool-down lessens the chance of injury. It does this by loosening the muscles and joints, raising and lowering the body temperature, and ensuring that the heart rate increases and then recovers, returning to its resting rate.

what is "warming up?"

Sometimes, due to lack of time or even just impatience, we leave out the most crucial stage of a workout—the warm-up. A thorough warm-up gradually prepares the body, both physically and mentally, for the more challenging physical activity—such as strength training or any form of aerobic activity—that is to follow.

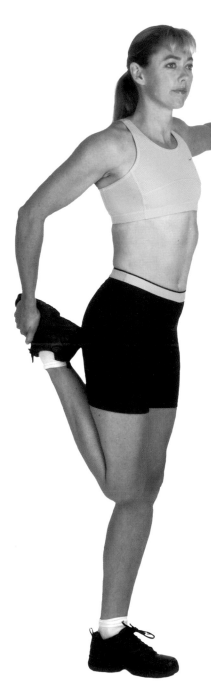

left: Gentle stretching of muscles is essential as part of your warm-up before strength training.

how to warm up

Warming up requires a minimum of five to ten minutes of gentle aerobic exercise, such as using an exercise bike, walking, or slow jogging on a treadmill, as preparation for strength training. When exercising at home or outdoors, a warm-up walk or gentle jog would be appropriate. This should be followed by some moderate stretching of the muscles that you will be using in your workout.

In colder weather your muscles tend to be stiffer and your body temperature is lower, so an increased warm-up time of fifteen to twenty minutes is recommended (thirty minutes in very cold climates).

benefits of warming up

• Increases the temperature within your muscles and tissue, thus decreasing muscle stiffness and lessening the chance of injury.

• Speeds up your heart rate, preparing your cardiovascular system for physical activity.

• Increases blood supply and oxygen uptake in the muscles that are being worked.

• Moves your body from a static to an active state, increasing awareness, arousal, mind/body coordination, and improving muscle response time to any movement.

• Mentally prepares you by clearing your mind, enabling you to focus on the workout.

• Improves range of movement and flexibility, allowing the muscles to move through a greater range of motion.

• Improves the production of various hormones, thus increasing the availability of carbohydrates and fatty acids for energy production.

what is "cooling down?"

The cool-down has the opposite effect of the warm-up, bringing your heart rate back to a resting level and helping your body to recover, relax, and prepare itself for its next activity.

This cooling-off period also prevents "blood pooling." When you work out, the heart is furiously pumping to supply oxygen-rich blood to the working muscle. By the end of your session, there may be an unusually large supply of blood left in the muscle. If this isn't returned swiftly back to the organs for central circulation, the brain may not receive an adequate amount of blood and you may start to feel dizzy and faint.

how to cool down

You should set aside five to ten minutes at the end of each exercise session for gentle stretching of the muscles worked. You should also include some light aerobic activity. Remember, in cold weather the cool-down should be around the same duration as the warm-up, about fifteen or twenty minutes (thirty minutes in a very cold climate).

benefits of cooling down

• Helps to return your heart rate, body temperature, and breathing to normal.

• Decreases any cramping or tightness felt in the muscles at rest or the following day.

• Reduces the risk of injury and dramatically increases flexibility, as the muscles are more supple and warm and can be stretched further with a greater increase in the range of movement after exercising.

• Removes any waste products (such as lactic acid) left behind in the muscles after exercising. This will reduce any potential muscle soreness that might occur after strength training.

If you still find that you are sore the next day, this means that lactic acid is still present in the muscle. Some gentle warm-up and cool-down exercises should help to ease any pain or discomfort felt at this time.

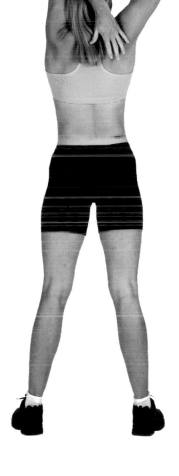

right and below: A good, slow stretch at the end of an exercise routine ensures that lactic acid isn't allowed to build up in your muscles, thereby preventing stiffness the next day.

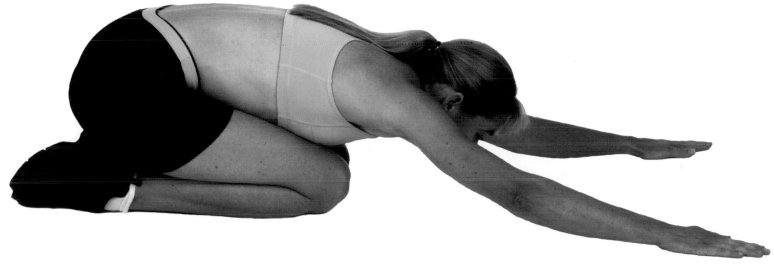

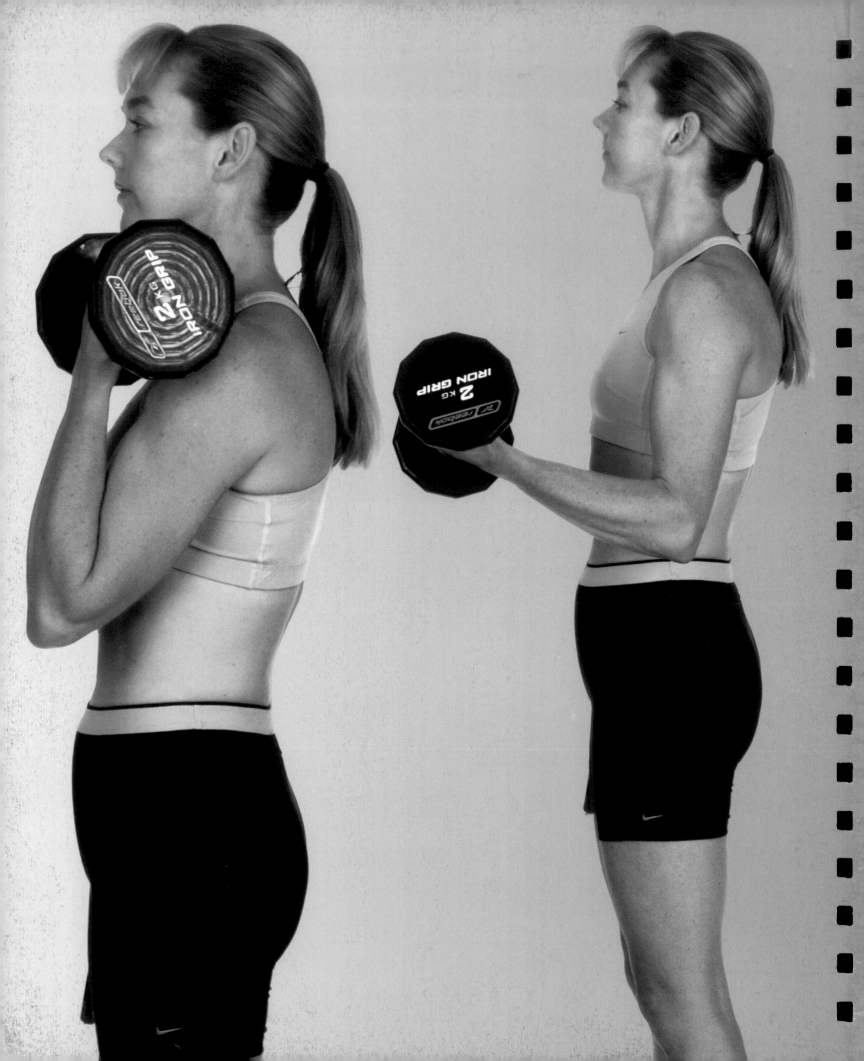

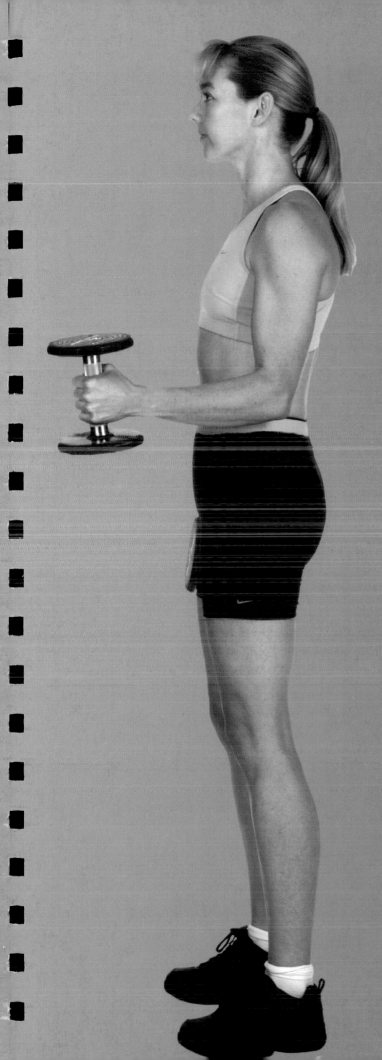

part 2

arms and
shoulders

shoulders

Also known as: musculus deltoideus, deltoids, delts

The deltoid is a large triangular muscle covering the shoulder joint and serving to abduct, flex, extend, and rotate the arm.

The shoulder muscle consists of the deltoid muscle, a large three-headed triangular muscle that originates from the clavicle and the scapula at the rear of the shoulder and extends down to the upper arm. The anterior deltoid functions to lift the arm to the front (as in front dumbbell raises, machine presses, barbell upright rows, and dumbbell presses). The medial deltoid serves to lift the arms to the side (as in dumbbell side raises). The posterior deltoid lifts the arms to the rear (as in bent-over dumbbell raises).

Since the deltoid is made up of three sections it is very important to work each area equally, to create an evenly toned and balanced shoulder muscle. Neglecting to work the area evenly can cause an imbalance within the muscle group—one area becomes stronger than another and the muscle is no longer able to work efficiently, which can lead to injury.

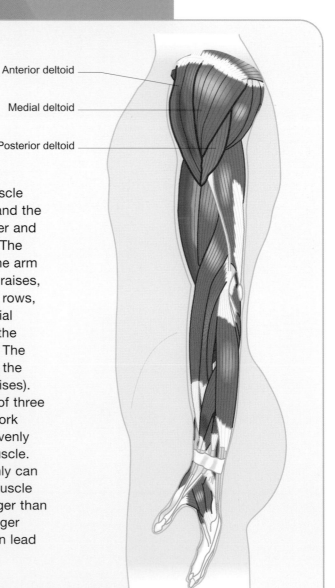

Anterior deltoid

Medial deltoid

Posterior deltoid

machine press (military press)

For the beginner who is unfamiliar with free weights or feels intimidated by them, this is the perfect machine. It allows you to improve your muscle coordination in the shoulder area in preparation for working with dumbbells.

level: beginner

main muscles worked: shoulders

secondary muscle worked: triceps

equipment used: machine press

type of exercise: size (mass) building

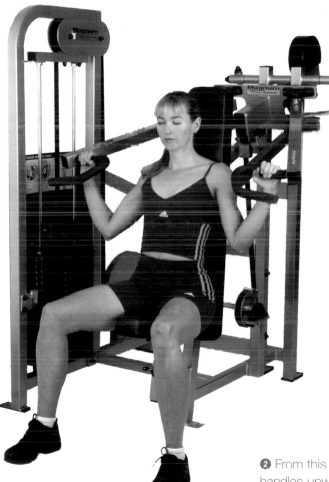

CAUTION

• Keep your elbows in position below your hands (without moving them outward as you lift and lower).

• Avoid bouncing the weight or letting it drop suddenly and slam down on the plate stack.

• Make sure the movement is smooth and controlled throughout.

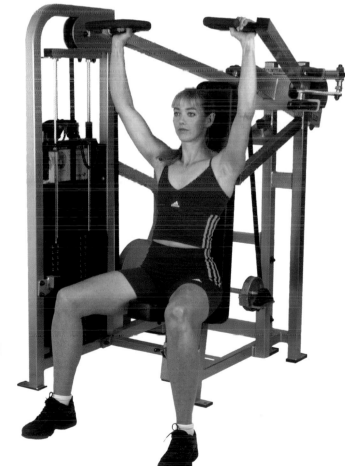

❶ First, adjust the seat so that the handles rest just above your shoulders. Make sure that your back is firmly against the back support, with your feet firmly on the ground in front of you, hip width apart. With your head up, looking straight ahead, place your hands on the handles with palms facing forward.

❷ From this position, push the handles upward over your head until your arms are extended (elbows slightly bent).

❸ In the raised position your arms should appear to be in a slight arc shape. Slowly lower the weight back down to the starting position (without letting the weight touch the stack) and repeat.

VARIATION

seated machine press (facing the backrest)

seated dumbbell press

This is one of the best free-weight exercises for building up the deltoid safely and effectively. The bench supports your body and a spotter (training companion) can take the weight off you if it becomes too heavy.

level: beginner
main muscles worked: shoulders
secondary muscles worked: triceps
equipment used: bench, dumbbells
type of exercise: size (mass)-building

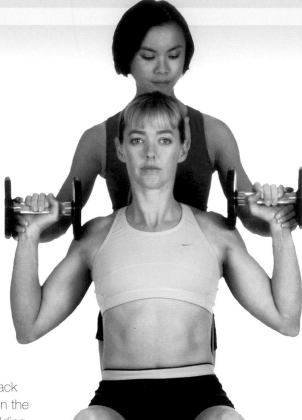

❶ Sit on an upright bench with a back support and place your feet firmly on the footrest or floor, hip width apart. Holding a dumbbell in each hand, position them on either side of your shoulders. Your elbows should be directly below your wrists with your palms facing forward. A spotter can stand behind you to ensure you are executing the exercise correctly and to take the weights if they become too heavy for you.

CAUTION

• Keep the movement smooth and even throughout and avoid bouncing the weights as you lift and lower.

• Make sure that your elbows remain slightly bent each time you raise upward and avoid thrusting your head forward.

• Keep your eyes focused straight ahead.

❷ From this position raise the dumbbells straight up above your head, keeping the movement smooth and controlled. Avoid lifting your shoulders as you raise the weight upward.

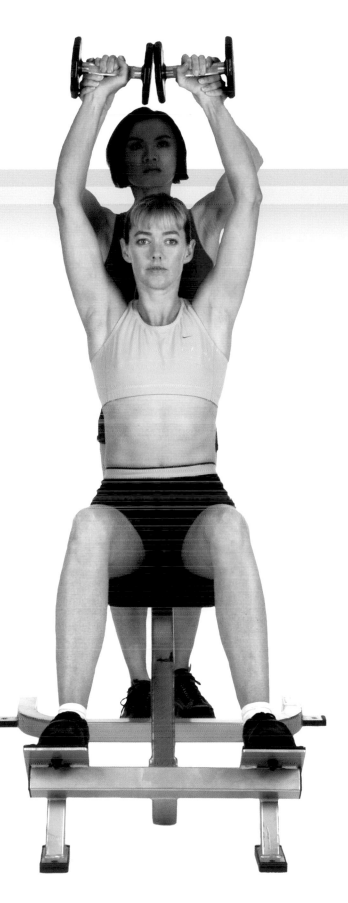

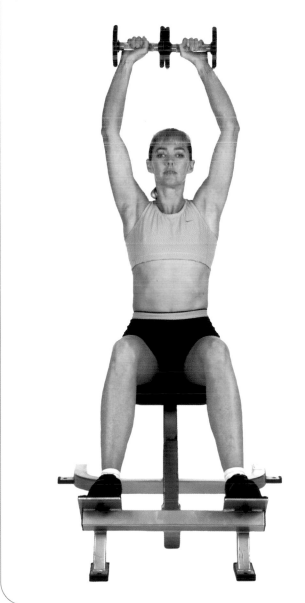

VARIATION

Once you have gained confidence in this exercise, you can perform the movement without the aid of a spotter.

❸ Continue raising the dumbbells until they are almost touching and your arms are extended (with your elbows very slightly bent), then slowly lower the dumbbells back to the starting position and repeat.

seated barbell military press

Once you have mastered the dumbbell and machine press, the next best free-weight exercise to attempt is the seated barbell military press. Although this exercise focuses on working the front of the shoulder (anterior delt), it will still work the whole of the shoulder area.

level: intermediate

main muscles worked: shoulders

secondary muscles worked: triceps

equipment used: bench, barbell

type of exercise: size (mass)-building

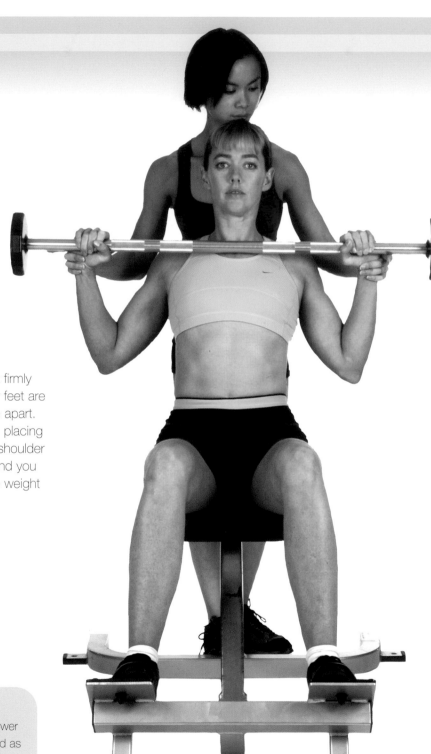

❶ Sit on an upright bench with your back firmly against the backrest. Make sure that your feet are firmly flat on the footrest or floor, hip width apart. Rest the barbell at the base of your neck, placing your hands on the bar slightly more than shoulder width apart. Have a spotter standing behind you to follow the movement, ready to take the weight from you if it becomes too much.

CAUTION
Avoid arching your back as you raise and lower the barbell. Also avoid leaning too far forward as you press the bar upward, which could cause you to lose your balance and injure yourself.

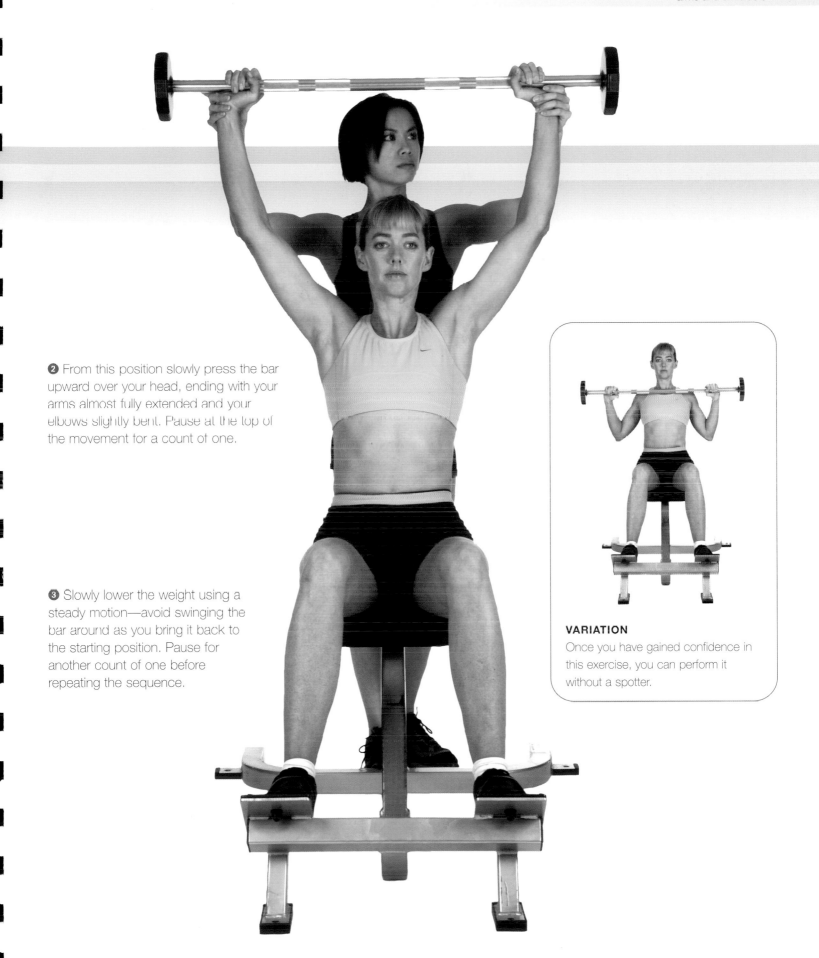

② From this position slowly press the bar upward over your head, ending with your arms almost fully extended and your elbows slightly bent. Pause at the top of the movement for a count of one.

③ Slowly lower the weight using a steady motion—avoid swinging the bar around as you bring it back to the starting position. Pause for another count of one before repeating the sequence.

VARIATION
Once you have gained confidence in this exercise, you can perform it without a spotter.

standing front dumbbell raise

This is an isolation exercise that specifically targets the intended muscle. The front raise will tone and shape the front of the shoulder (anterior deltoid), which helps define and separate the shoulder from the biceps and triceps.

level: beginner

main muscles worked: shoulders (specifically the front of the shoulder muscles—anterior deltoids)

secondary muscles worked: none

equipment used: dumbbells

type of exercise: isolation

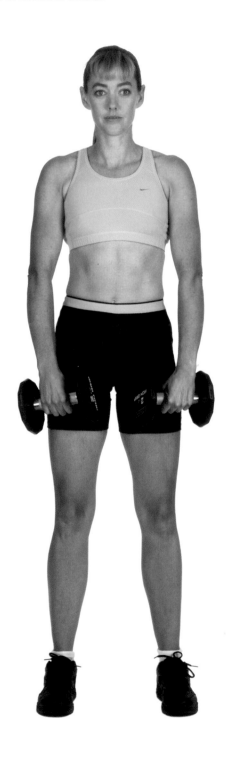

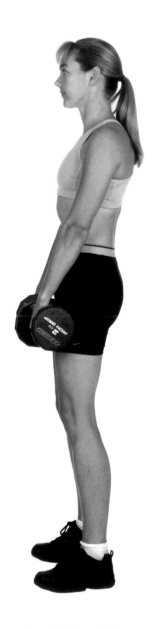

❶ Stand with your feet approximately hip width apart in front of a full-length mirror. Check that your legs are slightly bent and your back is straight. Keep your eyes facing forward, looking directly into the mirror. Hold the dumbbells, one in each hand, in front of you, resting them on your thighs, palms facing inward.

2 Keeping your arms extended and your elbows slightly bent, lift one arm in an arc formation, palm facing downward, raising the weight until it is at shoulder level.

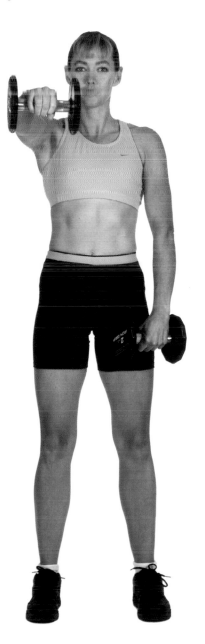

3 Pause in this position for a count of one. Then, using a smooth, controlled motion, lower the weight while simultaneously lifting the dumbbell in your other hand. Both arms should be in motion at the same time.

> **VARIATIONS**
>
> seated front raises, barbell front raises

CAUTION

• Stand tall with your back straight throughout and avoid hunching over as you lift and lower.

• Keep the movement slow and controlled and avoid cheating by swinging the weights, using your legs, or leaning backward.

• If you find that you cannot perform the exercise without cheating, then the weight is too heavy for you.

• An easier alternative to this movement is to raise and lower each arm in turn. For a more challenging version, raise and lower both arms together (making sure that you keep your shoulders dropped as you do so).

standing barbell upright rows

This is an excellent exercise for developing the shoulder muscle as well as the trapezius, and it helps to create separation between the shoulder and the chest muscle.

level: intermediate

main muscles worked: shoulders (specifically the front and side—anterior and medial deltoids)

secondary muscles worked: biceps, trapezius

equipment used: barbell

type of exercise: size (mass)-building

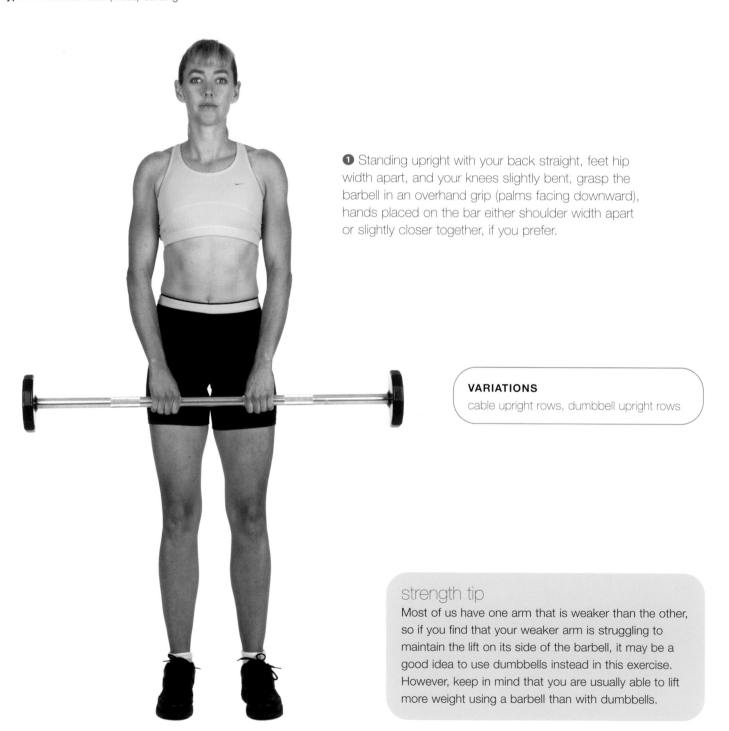

❶ Standing upright with your back straight, feet hip width apart, and your knees slightly bent, grasp the barbell in an overhand grip (palms facing downward), hands placed on the bar either shoulder width apart or slightly closer together, if you prefer.

VARIATIONS

cable upright rows, dumbbell upright rows

strength tip

Most of us have one arm that is weaker than the other, so if you find that your weaker arm is struggling to maintain the lift on its side of the barbell, it may be a good idea to use dumbbells instead in this exercise. However, keep in mind that you are usually able to lift more weight using a barbell than with dumbbells.

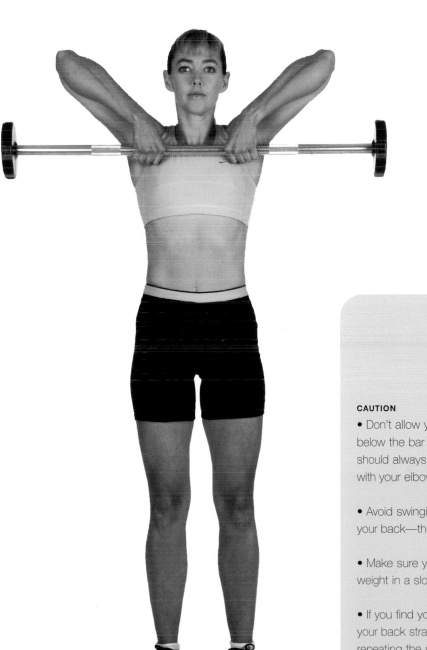

❷ Raise the barbell upward, keeping the bar level with and as close to your body as possible. As you raise the bar, make sure that you lead the movement with your elbows, keeping them lifted higher than your hands throughout. Your shoulders should remain dropped as you raise the bar.

❸ Keep raising the bar until it is at chest level, then without pausing, slowly lower the weight back to the starting position. Repeat.

CAUTION

• Don't allow your elbows to drop below the bar (as pictured here). You should always lead the movement with your elbows higher than the bar.

• Avoid swinging the bar or arching your back—these can cause injury.

• Make sure you raise and lower the weight in a slow, controlled manner.

• If you find yourself unable to keep your back straight as you work, try repeating the sequence leaning up against a wall or post to help keep your back flat and straight.

machine side raises

This machine allows the beginner to exercise her deltoid muscle with little danger of injuring herself or performing the exercise incorrectly.

level: beginner

main muscles worked: shoulders (specifically the sides of the shoulder muscles—medial delts)

secondary muscles worked: none

equipment used: side raise machine

type of exercise: isolation

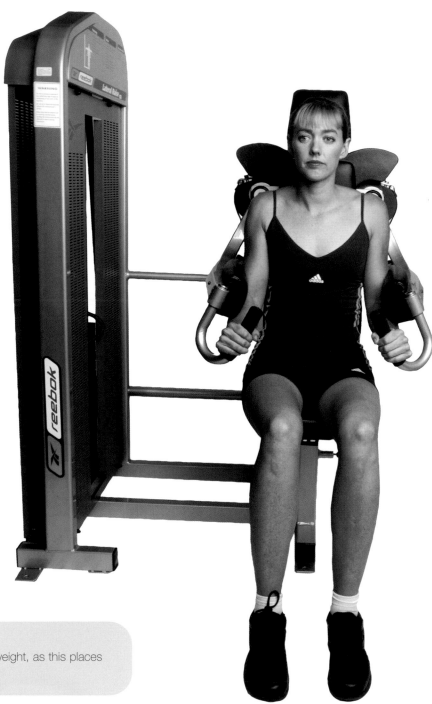

❶ Adjust the seat so that you can place your feet firmly on the floor. Position yourself so that your back is comfortably supported by the backrest. Grasp the handlebars, making sure the side pads are pressed up against your upper arms between your elbows and shoulder region.

CAUTION
Avoid arching your back while lifting the weight, as this places unnecessary stress on your lower back.

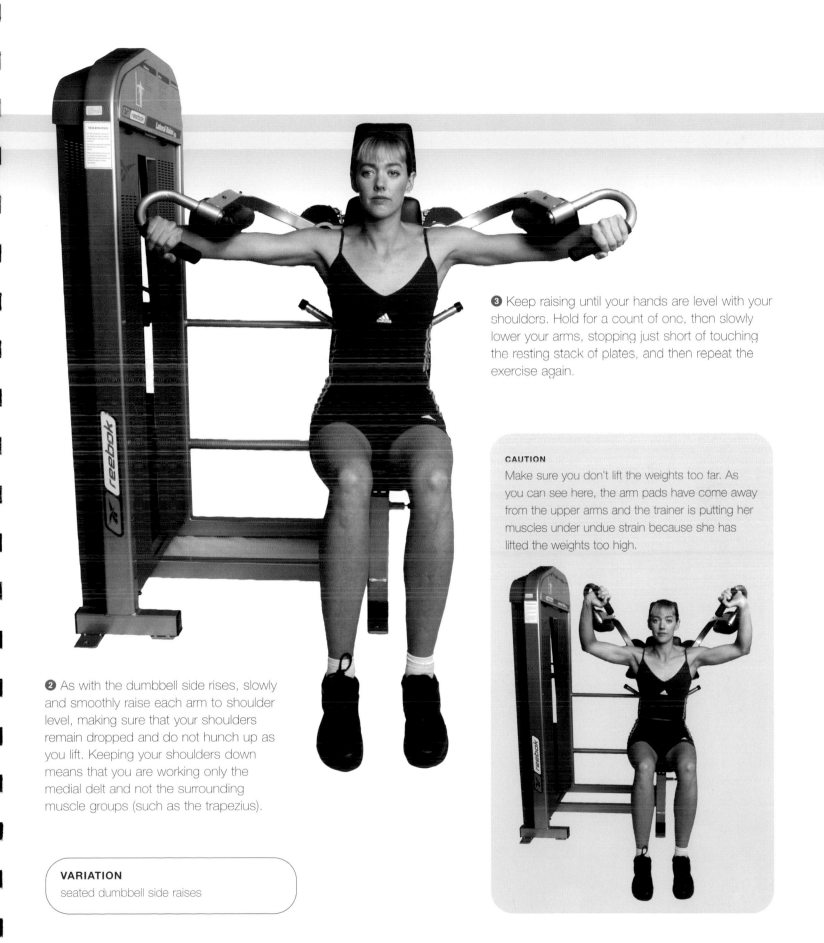

❸ Keep raising until your hands are level with your shoulders. Hold for a count of one, then slowly lower your arms, stopping just short of touching the resting stack of plates, and then repeat the exercise again.

CAUTION

Make sure you don't lift the weights too far. As you can see here, the arm pads have come away from the upper arms and the trainer is putting her muscles under undue strain because she has lifted the weights too high.

❷ As with the dumbbell side rises, slowly and smoothly raise each arm to shoulder level, making sure that your shoulders remain dropped and do not hunch up as you lift. Keeping your shoulders down means that you are working only the medial delt and not the surrounding muscle groups (such as the trapezius).

VARIATION
seated dumbbell side raises

seated dumbbell side raises

This is a great exercise for shaping and toning the side of the shoulder, separating the muscle from other muscle groups on the arm (the triceps and biceps). Lateral raises create a more rounded and defined look to the shoulder.

level: intermediate

main muscles worked: shoulders (specifically the sides of the shoulder muscles—medial delts)

secondary muscles worked: none

equipment used: bench, dumbbells

type of exercise: isolation

❶ Sit on an upright bench, placing your feet firmly on the footrest or floor, hip width apart. Your arms should be at your sides, with a dumbbell in each hand, and your palms should be facing your thighs.

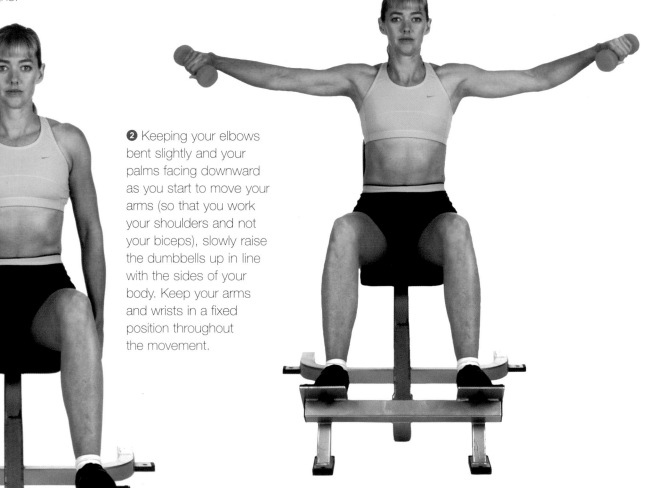

❷ Keeping your elbows bent slightly and your palms facing downward as you start to move your arms (so that you work your shoulders and not your biceps), slowly raise the dumbbells up in line with the sides of your body. Keep your arms and wrists in a fixed position throughout the movement.

❸ Continue lifting your arms slowly upward until the weights are at shoulder level, tilting your hands forward slightly as you reach this position so that your little fingers are raised fractionally higher than your thumbs (to fully isolate the deltoid muscle). Hold this position for a count of one, then slowly lower to the starting position and repeat the movement.

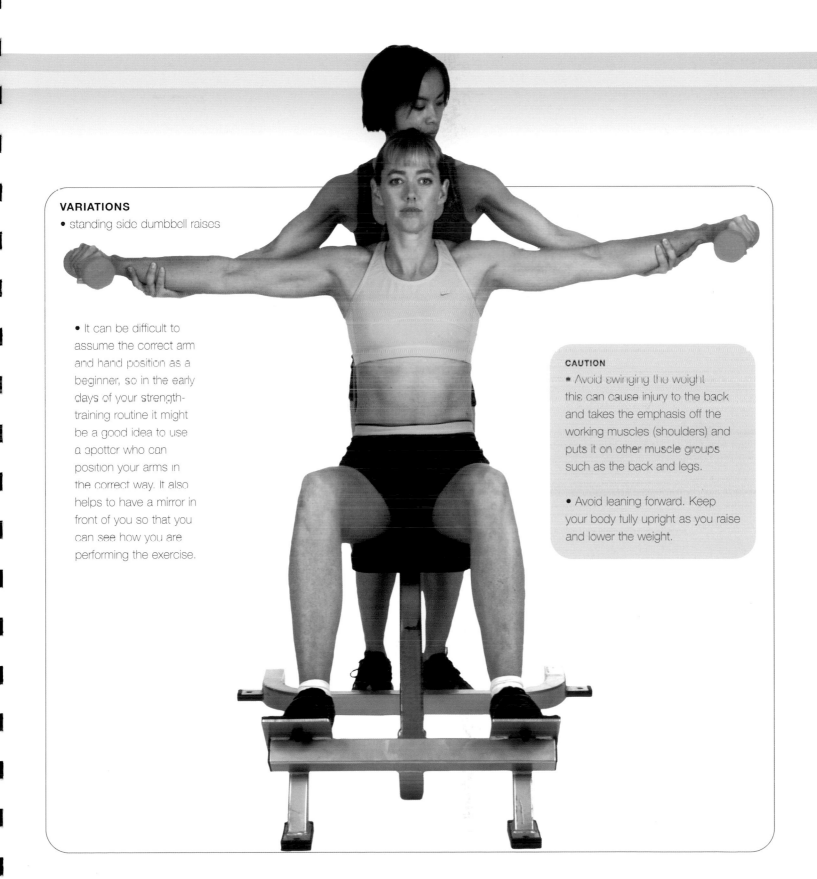

VARIATIONS

• standing side dumbbell raises

• It can be difficult to assume the correct arm and hand position as a beginner, so in the early days of your strength-training routine it might be a good idea to use a spotter who can position your arms in the correct way. It also helps to have a mirror in front of you so that you can see how you are performing the exercise.

CAUTION

• Avoid swinging the weight: this can cause injury to the back and takes the emphasis off the working muscles (shoulders) and puts it on other muscle groups such as the back and legs.

• Avoid leaning forward. Keep your body fully upright as you raise and lower the weight.

seated bent-over rear dumbbell raises

This exercise is great for strengthening the back of the shoulder muscles (posterior delts). For those who suffer from bad posture or rounded shoulders, it encourages you to bring your shoulders back and helps you develop sufficient strength to stand taller and straighter.

level: intermediate

main muscles worked: shoulders (specifically the rear section of the shoulder muscles—posterior delts)

secondary muscles worked: none

equipment used: bench, dumbbells

type of exercise: isolation

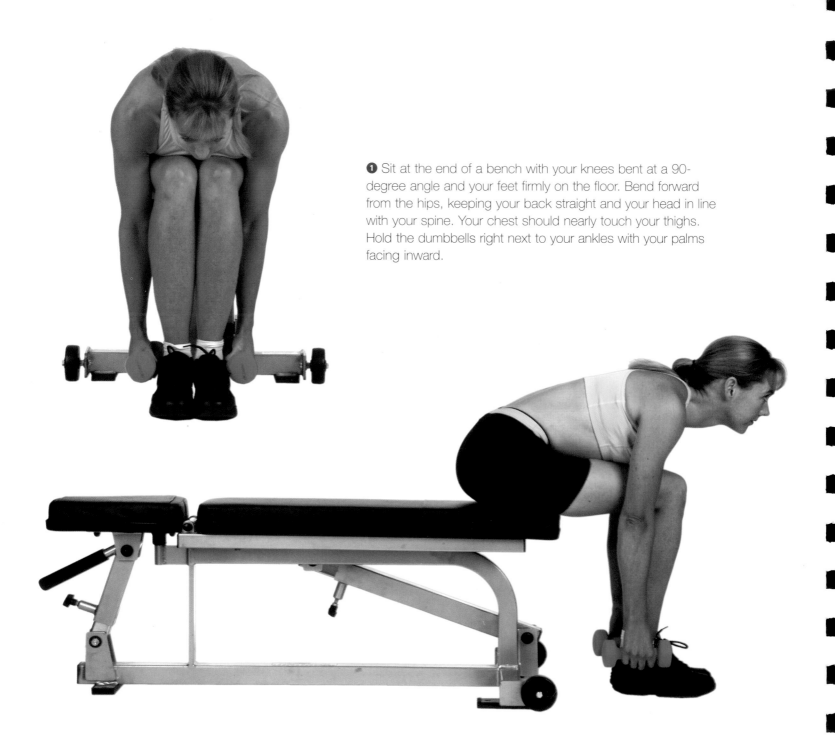

❶ Sit at the end of a bench with your knees bent at a 90-degree angle and your feet firmly on the floor. Bend forward from the hips, keeping your back straight and your head in line with your spine. Your chest should nearly touch your thighs. Hold the dumbbells right next to your ankles with your palms facing inward.

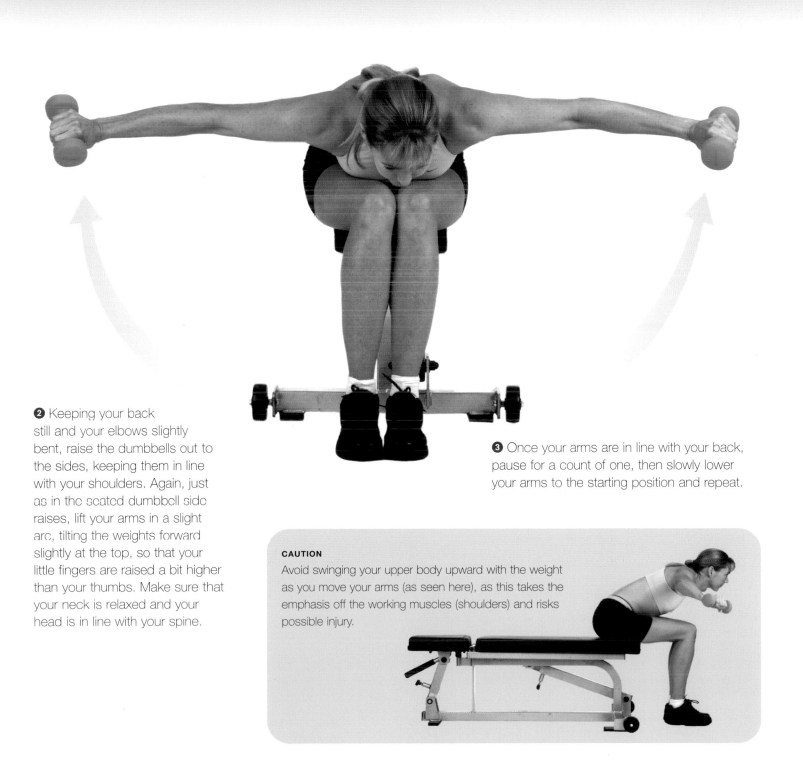

❷ Keeping your back still and your elbows slightly bent, raise the dumbbells out to the sides, keeping them in line with your shoulders. Again, just as in the seated dumbbell side raises, lift your arms in a slight arc, tilting the weights forward slightly at the top, so that your little fingers are raised a bit higher than your thumbs. Make sure that your neck is relaxed and your head is in line with your spine.

❸ Once your arms are in line with your back, pause for a count of one, then slowly lower your arms to the starting position and repeat.

CAUTION
Avoid swinging your upper body upward with the weight as you move your arms (as seen here), as this takes the emphasis off the working muscles (shoulders) and risks possible injury.

machine reverse pec deck

This is a fixed-weight alternative to the supported rear dumbbell raises for the backs of the shoulders (posterior delts) and is ideal for those who are having difficulty with the bent-over rear dumbbell raises. This sequence places you in a comfortable position with your back fully supported.

level: intermediate

main muscles worked: shoulders (specifically the rear—posterior delts)

secondary muscles worked: none

equipment used: reverse pec deck machine

type of exercise: isolation

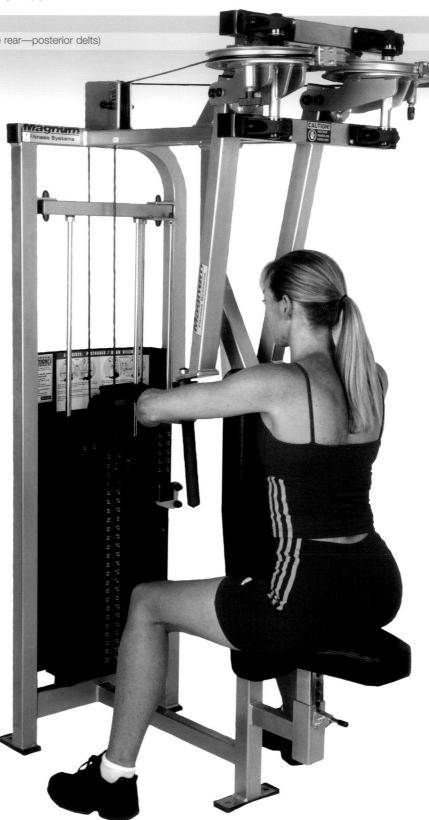

❶ Adjust the seat so that you can place your feet firmly on the floor approximately hip width apart. Adjust the machine handles so that they are positioned right in front of you. Sit firmly in the seat and grasp the handles with your palms facing toward you.

❷ Focus your eyes straight ahead, then slowly open your arms outward (keeping your elbows slightly bent) and bring them back in line with the rest of your body.

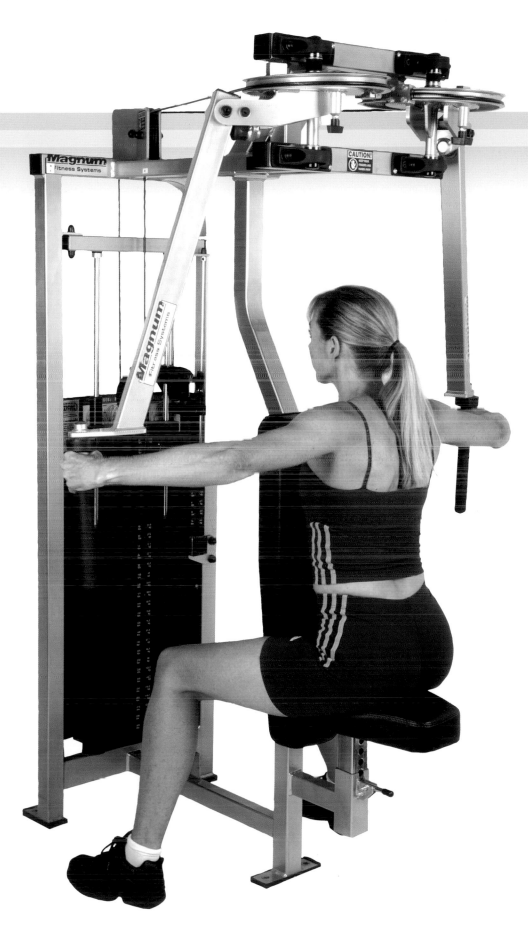

❸ Pause for a count of one, then slowly return to the starting position, making sure that the weight doesn't touch the plate stack. Repeat.

CAUTION

• Make sure the exercise is carried out using a slow, continuous, and controlled movement.

• Avoid slamming the weights together at the start position. This can cause unnecessary jolting and strain to the shoulder muscle.

bench-supported rear dumbbell raises

This exercise has the same effect as the seated bent-over rear dumbbell raises; it's a good alternative for those who need extra back support.

level: intermediate

main muscles worked: shoulders (specifically the rear part of the shoulder—posterior delt)

secondary muscles worked: none

equipment used: incline bench, dumbbells

type of exercise: isolation

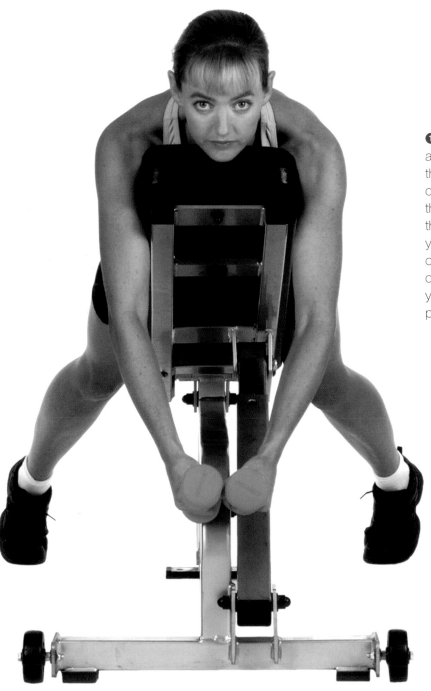

❶ Set the incline bench backrest at a 45-degree angle. The backrest should be facing away from the mirror (if there is one in the gym). Lie facedown on the bench with your head just over the top of the backrest (your chin should rest on the top of the bench). Your legs should be slightly bent, with your feet resting on the floor. Grasp the dumbbells, one in each hand, with your palms facing each other. Keeping your elbows slightly bent, extend your arms down in front of you so that they are perpendicular to the angle of the bench.

CAUTION

• Avoid raising your head up as you move your arms—this can place unwanted stress on your neck vertebrae.

• Keep your upper body in contact with the bench throughout; lifting up as you move your arms can place unnecessary stress on your neck muscles.

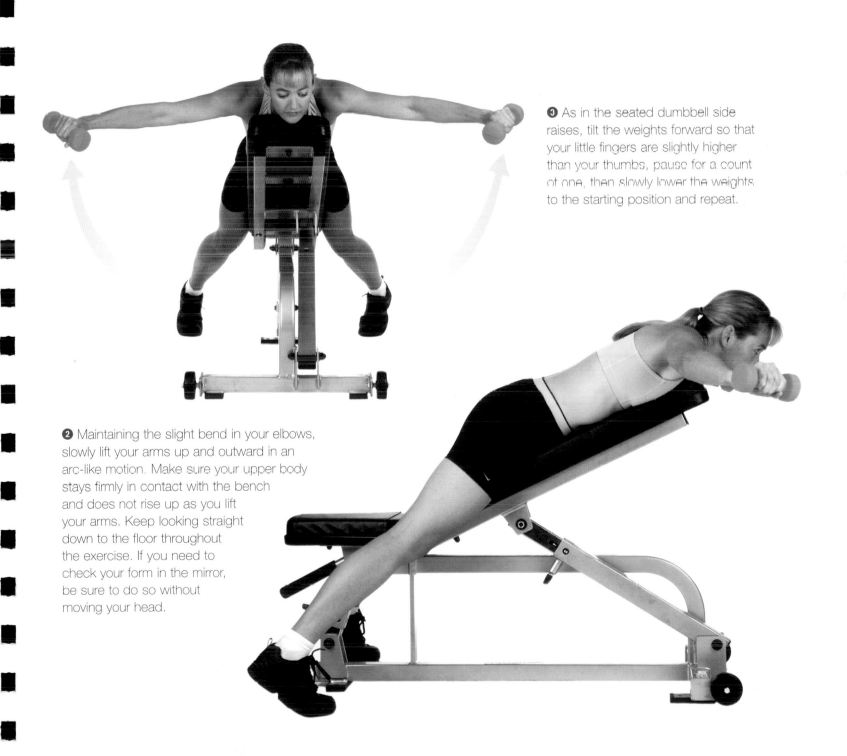

3 As in the seated dumbbell side raises, tilt the weights forward so that your little fingers are slightly higher than your thumbs, pause for a count of one, then slowly lower the weights to the starting position and repeat.

2 Maintaining the slight bend in your elbows, slowly lift your arms up and outward in an arc-like motion. Make sure your upper body stays firmly in contact with the bench and does not rise up as you lift your arms. Keep looking straight down to the floor throughout the exercise. If you need to check your form in the mirror, be sure to do so without moving your head.

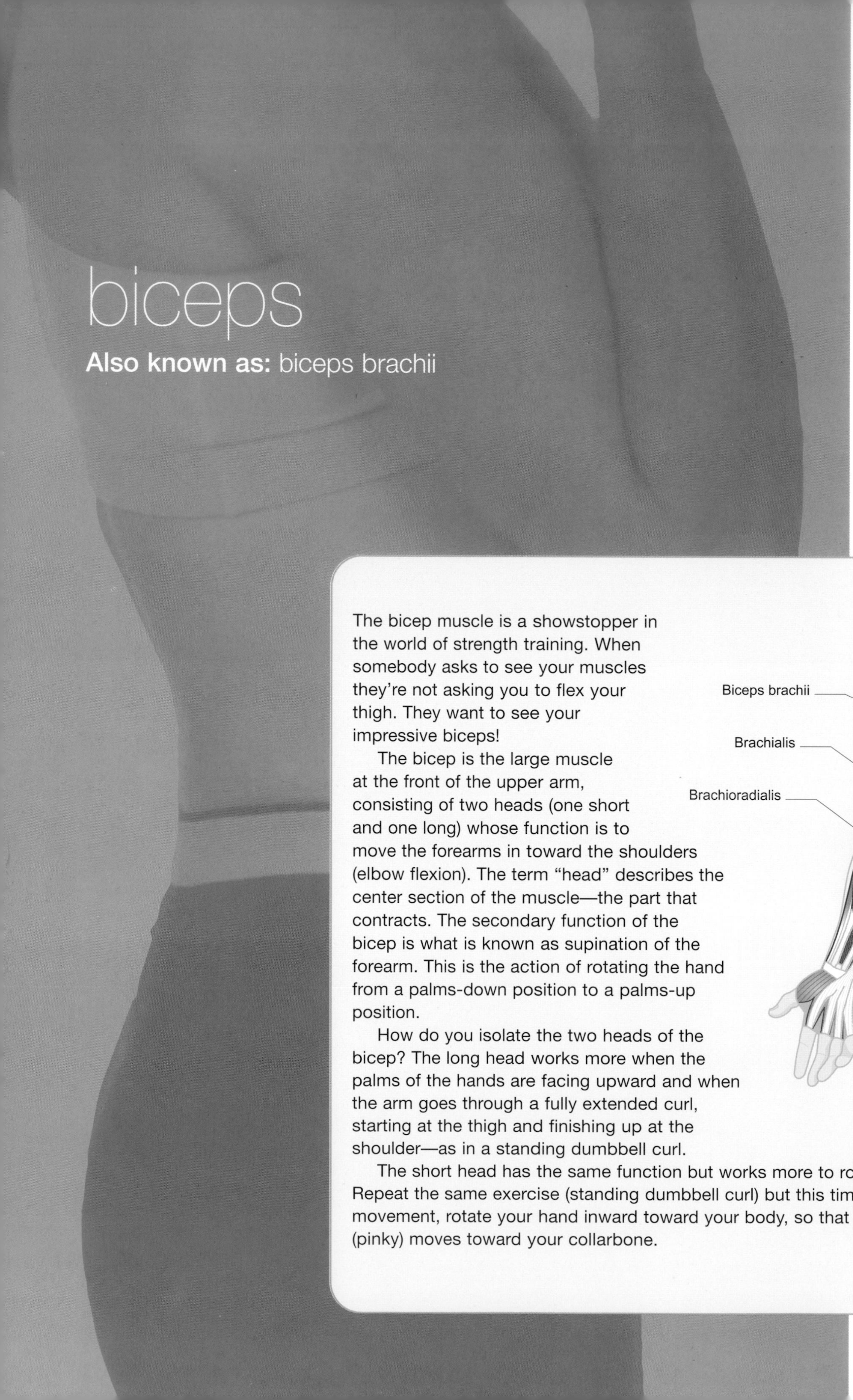

biceps

Also known as: biceps brachii

The bicep muscle is a showstopper in the world of strength training. When somebody asks to see your muscles they're not asking you to flex your thigh. They want to see your impressive biceps!

The bicep is the large muscle at the front of the upper arm, consisting of two heads (one short and one long) whose function is to move the forearms in toward the shoulders (elbow flexion). The term "head" describes the center section of the muscle—the part that contracts. The secondary function of the bicep is what is known as supination of the forearm. This is the action of rotating the hand from a palms-down position to a palms-up position.

How do you isolate the two heads of the bicep? The long head works more when the palms of the hands are facing upward and when the arm goes through a fully extended curl, starting at the thigh and finishing up at the shoulder—as in a standing dumbbell curl.

The short head has the same function but works more to rotate the forearm. Repeat the same exercise (standing dumbbell curl) but this time, at the end of the movement, rotate your hand inward toward your body, so that your little finger (pinky) moves toward your collarbone.

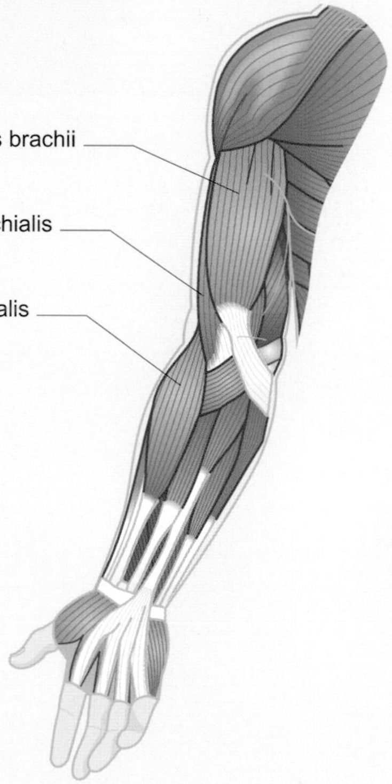

Biceps brachii

Brachialis

Brachioradialis

standing barbell curls

This exercise is considered to be one of the best and most effective for giving some size and shape to the upper arms (biceps). It is an easy exercise to master for those who have done no previous training for their bicep muscles.

level: beginner
main muscles worked: biceps
secondary muscles worked: forearms
equipment used: barbell
type of exercise: size (mass)-building

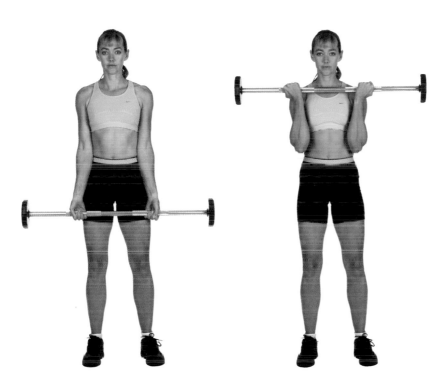

CAUTION

• Avoid swinging backward or forward as you lift and lower; this can cause you to lose your balance and risks injury to your back.

• Check that your hands are the correct distance apart and that your handgrip is neither too narrow nor too wide—both of these can cause stress and strain to the wrists and elbows.

• Don't allow the bar to tip at one end or the other. Throughout the movement, the barbell should be held evenly horizontal to the floor.

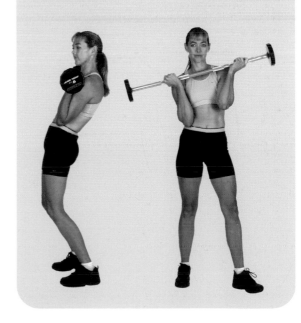

❶ Stand with your feet approximately hip width apart and your toes turned slightly outward for balance. Check that your knees are slightly bent and your back is straight. Keeping your elbows slightly bent and tucked in to your sides, grasp the barbell with your hands roughly shoulder width apart and your palms facing away from you.

❷ Avoiding swaying or swinging forward with the bar; use one slow, continuous movement to bring the bar in toward your shoulders, keeping your elbows tight to your sides. Avoid the temptation of moving your whole arm away from your body as you lift the weight up and out—this action would take the focus off the bicep, the muscle you are trying to work.

❸ Bring the barbell in until it is level with the top of your chest, just below your chin. Hold for a count of one, squeezing the bicep muscle to maximize the effectiveness of the exercise, and then lower to the starting position. If you are unsure how to squeeze the muscle, just imagine you have an orange between your bicep and forearm that you are trying to squeeze.

standing dumbbell curls

This is an alternative to the standing barbell curls and is good for those who suffer from wrist pain or discomfort when holding their hands in a fixed position.

level: beginner

main muscles worked: biceps

secondary muscles worked: forearms

equipment used: dumbbells

type of exercise: size (mass)-building

❶ Holding the dumbbells by your sides, palms facing inward, stand with your back straight, looking straight ahead. Your feet should be placed approximately hip width apart, with your toes turned slightly outward for balance.

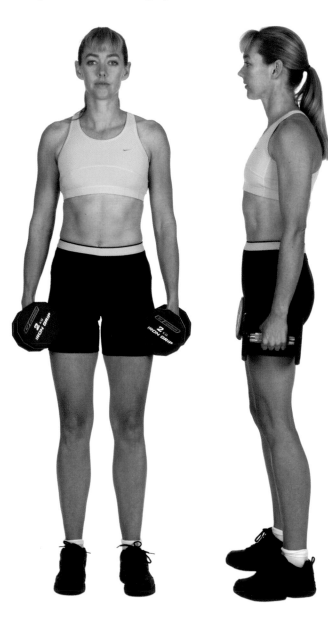

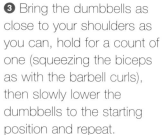

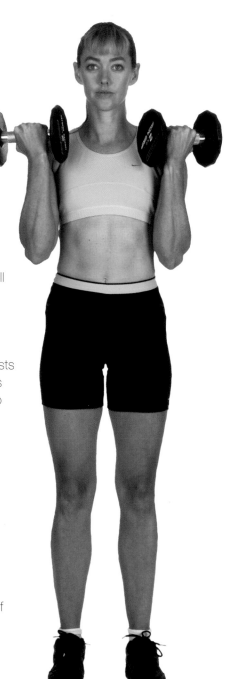

❷ As in the standing barbell curl, make sure you avoid swaying or leaning too far forward. Slowly curl the dumbbells in toward your shoulders, rotating your wrists upward once your forearms are at a 90-degree angle to your body. Make sure that your elbows remain firmly tucked in to your sides throughout this exercise.

❸ Bring the dumbbells as close to your shoulders as you can, hold for a count of one (squeezing the biceps as with the barbell curls), then slowly lower the dumbbells to the starting position and repeat.

strength tip

You may find that one arm, or one side of the body, is stronger than the other. Don't worry; this is quite common. Using dumbbells instead of a barbell is a great way of making each arm work independently, allowing the body to balance itself and develop equal strength on both sides.

VARIATION

This exercise can be done alternating the arms (raising one arm while you lower the other) instead of moving them both together.

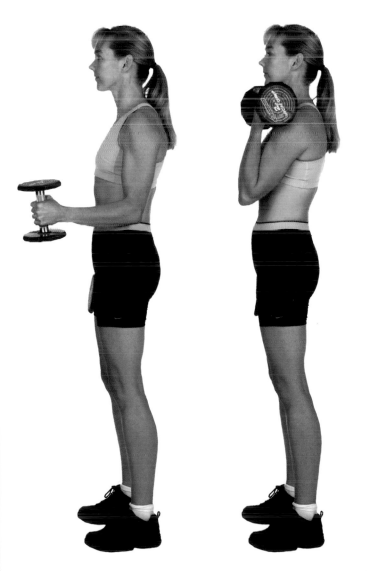

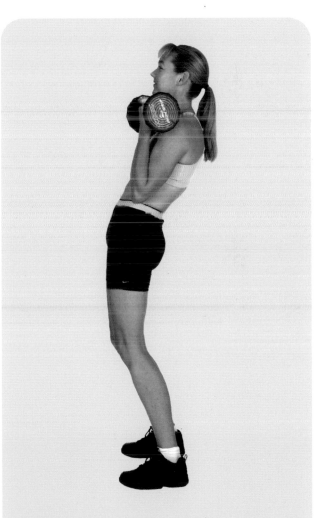

CAUTION

It is very easy to cheat with this exercise, using an incorrect technique to lift or lower the weight. Just remember that it is not a race; keep the movement slow and controlled as you lift and lower your forearms and rotate your wrists. You will gain much more benefit from performing this exercise correctly than if you hurry to finish and risk injuring yourself.

seated dumbbell curls

This version of dumbbell curls is an excellent alternative for those who suffer from back problems and need the extra support of a backrest. It's also good for those who find it uncomfortable to stand while doing bicep exercises.

level: beginner

main muscles worked: biceps

secondary muscles worked: none

equipment used: bench, dumbbells

type of exercise: size (mass)-building

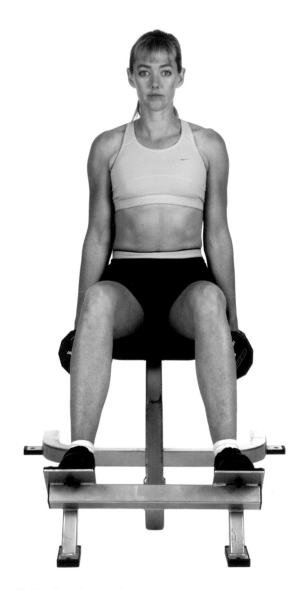

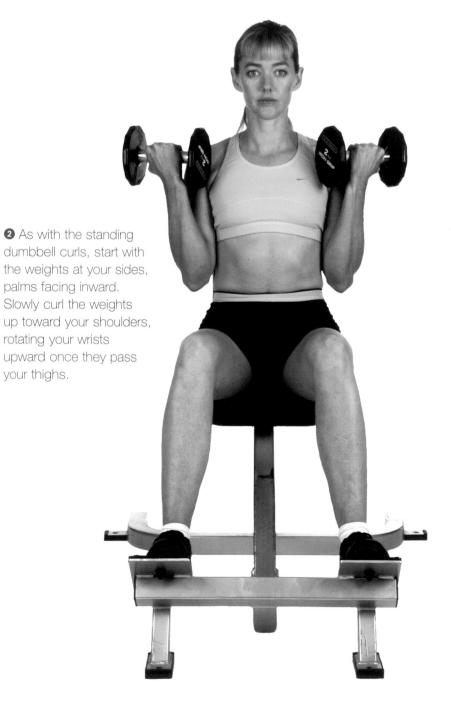

❷ As with the standing dumbbell curls, start with the weights at your sides, palms facing inward. Slowly curl the weights up toward your shoulders, rotating your wrists upward once they pass your thighs.

❶ Position the backrest so that it is fully upright (at a 90-degree angle), then sit facing forward, looking straight into the mirror with your head up. Place your feet on the footrest or floor about hip width apart.

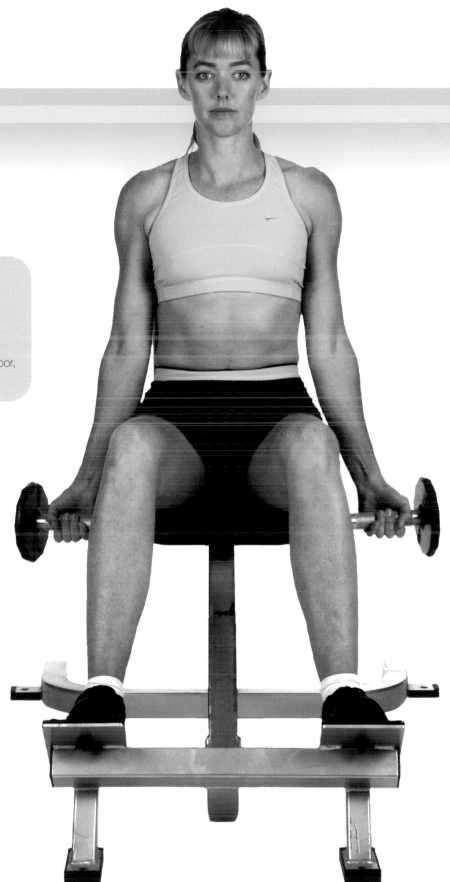

CAUTION

• Keep your elbows tucked in to your sides throughout the exercise.

• Make sure that you keep your eyes focused straight ahead, rather than looking down at the floor, which places unwanted stress on your neck.

❸ Bring the dumbbells as close as you can to your shoulders, keeping your palms facing inward. Squeeze the biceps while holding the weight for a count of one, then slowly lower to the starting position and repeat the movement.

standing hammer dumbbell curls

The principles for the standing dumbbell and barbell curls also apply here. The only difference is that your palms face toward each other throughout the entire movement.

level: beginner
main muscles worked: biceps
secondary muscles worked: forearms
equipment used: dumbbells
type of exercise: isolation

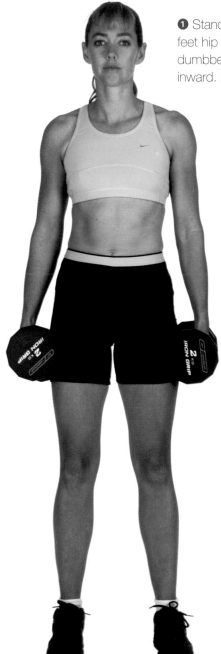

❶ Stand tall with your back straight and your feet hip width apart, arms at your sides, a dumbbell in each hand, and your palms facing inward. Focus your eyes straight ahead.

❷ Keeping your elbows tucked in to your sides, lift the weights up toward your shoulders, palms facing inward. Only your forearms should move; your upper arms and elbows should remain stationary throughout the entire sequence.

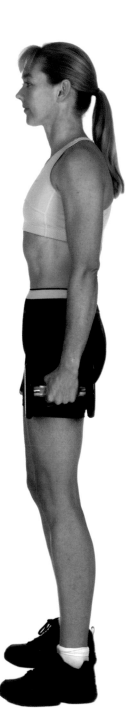

strength tip

To perform the hammer curls correctly, imagine that you are copying the action of hammering a nail into a piece of wood—hence the name. This movement may be a little easier to learn than the standing dumbbell and barbell curls, as there is no upward twisting of the wrist, just a simple up-and-down motion.

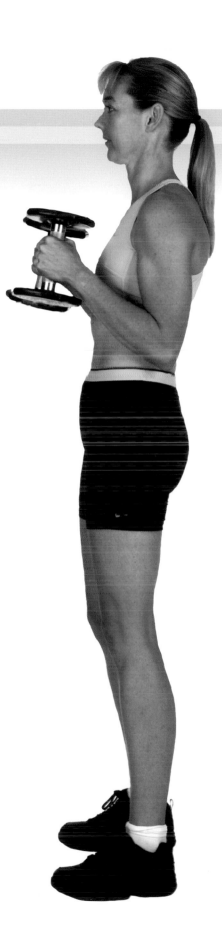

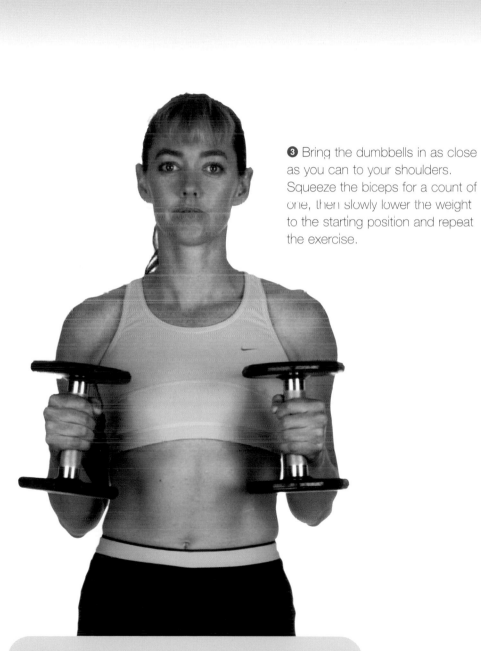

❸ Bring the dumbbells in as close as you can to your shoulders. Squeeze the biceps for a count of one, then slowly lower the weight to the starting position and repeat the exercise.

CAUTION

• Keep your elbows tucked in to your sides throughout the movement.

• Keep your eyes focused straight ahead rather than looking downward, which would place unwanted stress on your neck.

seated machine bicep curls

The machine curls are a great alternative if you have problems mastering the dumbbells, and they also add variety to your routine. However, this exercise does restrict the natural movement of your arms, since they remain in a fixed position from start to finish.

level: beginner

main muscles worked: biceps

secondary muscles worked: forearms

equipment used: bicep curl machine

type of exercise: isolation

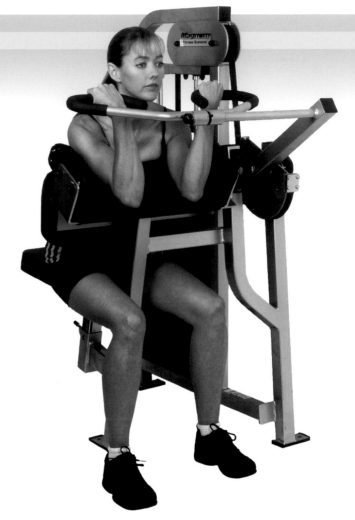

❶ Adjust the seat so that you can place your feet firmly on the floor with your knees at a 90-degree angle. You should be able to rest the back of your upper arm comfortably on the machine pad without having to lean over the pad too far. Keeping your elbows slightly bent, grasp the machine handles, palms facing toward you, thumbs on the grip.

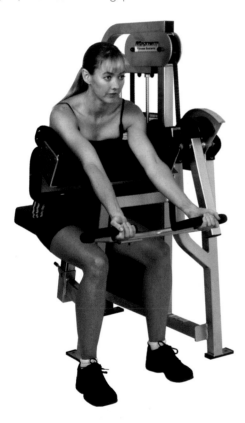

❷ Bring the handlebars up toward your shoulders as far as you can, lifting the weight in a slow, controlled manner. If you find that you are rocking your body forward or swinging to move the weight toward you, the weight is probably too heavy for you. The goal is to make the exercise hard enough to allow you to feel your biceps working, but not so hard that it becomes difficult to move the weight.

CAUTION

• Do not bounce, jerk, or swing your body backward or forward to move the weight from start to finish; this will only cause injury to the bicep muscle.

• If possible, always choose a weight that you can comfortably lift for at least twelve repetitions.

❸ As with most bicep exercises, raise your hands until they are level with the front of your shoulders. Hold for a count of one and squeeze your biceps, then slowly lower your arms to the starting position. Stop the movement just short of fully extending your arms, making sure you don't allow the weight to touch the plate stack. This ensures that continuous tension is maintained on the working muscles (the biceps).

standing one-arm dumbbell curl over bench

This exercise isolates the lower part of the bicep (the long head). It creates length and a bulge in the bicep. It also helps to separate the bicep from the forearm, so the muscle seems to stand alone rather than blending into the rest of the arm.

level: intermediate

main muscles worked: biceps

secondary muscles worked: forearms

equipment used: incline bench, dumbbell

type of exercise: isolation

❶ Stand behind an incline bench with the backrest at a little less than a 90-degree angle. Place your feet approximately hip width apart with your knees slightly bent. To help you balance you may want to place one foot slightly behind the other one, as in a lunge or walking stance. Bend forward from your hips, keeping your back straight. Avoid hunching over the bench, which can cause unwanted strain on your lower back. Holding a dumbbell in one hand, extend your arm, palm up, with your upper arm and elbow on the bench, elbow slightly bent.

❷ Keeping the rest of your body still, curl the dumbbell up toward your shoulder until your forearm touches your bicep. If you find yourself needing to twist your body or move your shoulder in order to lift the weight, the dumbbell is probably too heavy for you.

❸ Raise the dumbbell until it is just in front of your shoulder. Squeeze the bicep for a count of one, then slowly lower the dumbbell to the starting position and repeat. Do at least twelve repetitions on one arm and then switch position and repeat the sequence for the other arm.

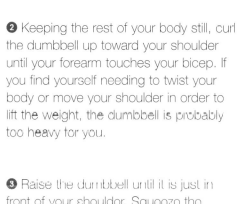

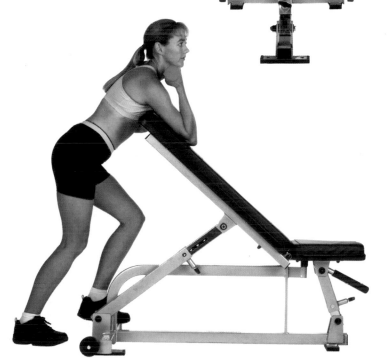

CAUTION

Keep your upper arm in contact with the bench to maintain the tension in the muscle you are trying to work (the bicep). Raise and lower the weight in a slow, controlled manner.

seated dumbbell concentration curls

As with all bicep exercises, this one offers another way of working the bicep muscle from yet another angle. As well as improving shape and definition, the concentration curl helps create a peak to the bicep, so that when you flex, there is a pronounced shape to the muscle.

level: intermediate
main muscles worked: biceps
secondary muscles worked: forearms
equipment used: bench, dumbbell
type of exercise: isolation

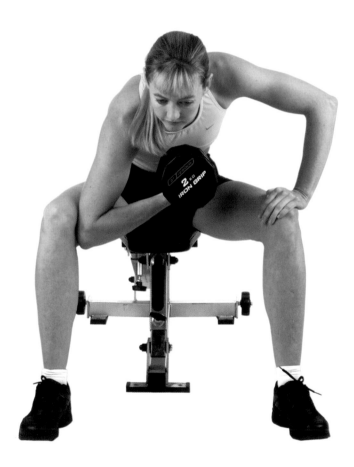

CAUTION
The golden rule: if you find you're using other muscle groups or the rest of your body to lift the weight, it's too heavy! Just remember, strength will come in time. Avoid rushing or you risk causing yourself an injury.

❸ Hold for a count of one at the top and squeeze your bicep, then lower the weight to the original position with your arm extended, using a slow, controlled movement. Complete your desired number of reps and sets on this arm, then switch position and repeat for the other arm.

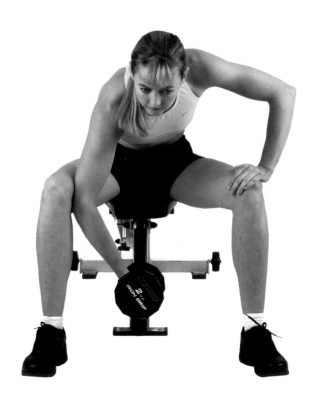

❶ Sit on the end of a flat bench with your legs apart in a V shape and your toes turned slightly outward. Lean over toward your thighs, keeping your back straight. Rest your right elbow on the inside of your right thigh while holding a dumbbell, palm facing toward the opposite leg. Extend your right arm, keeping the elbow slightly bent. Rest your left hand or forearm on your left thigh for support.

❷ Keeping your upper arm firmly against your thigh, lift the weight up toward your shoulder. Avoid moving your upper body or shoulder as you raise the weight.

standing two-arm cable curls

This exercise is similar to the standing barbell curls and standing dumbbell curls, but it uses handle attachments. A little more coordination, control, and understanding is required. You can use quite a bit of forearm rotation to vary the movement.

level: intermediate

main muscles worked: biceps

secondary muscles worked: forearms

equipment used: two handles on a cable machine

type of exercise: size (mass)-building

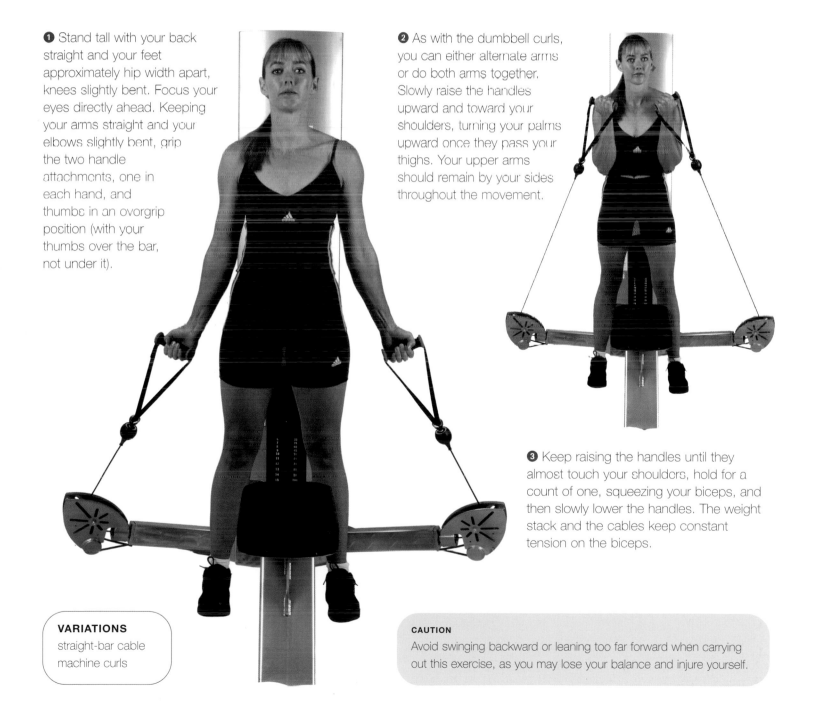

❶ Stand tall with your back straight and your feet approximately hip width apart, knees slightly bent. Focus your eyes directly ahead. Keeping your arms straight and your elbows slightly bent, grip the two handle attachments, one in each hand, and thumbs in an overgrip position (with your thumbs over the bar, not under it).

❷ As with the dumbbell curls, you can either alternate arms or do both arms together. Slowly raise the handles upward and toward your shoulders, turning your palms upward once they pass your thighs. Your upper arms should remain by your sides throughout the movement.

❸ Keep raising the handles until they almost touch your shoulders, hold for a count of one, squeezing your biceps, and then slowly lower the handles. The weight stack and the cables keep constant tension on the biceps.

VARIATIONS
straight-bar cable machine curls

CAUTION
Avoid swinging backward or leaning too far forward when carrying out this exercise, as you may lose your balance and injure yourself.

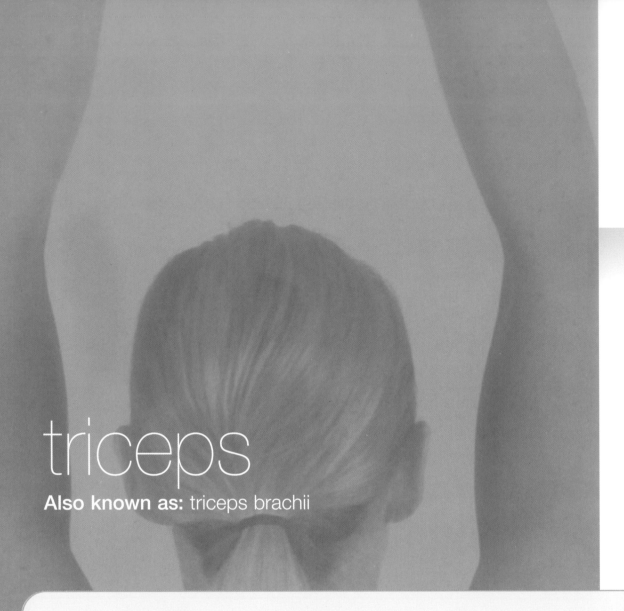

triceps

Also known as: triceps brachii

The tricep is a large horseshoe-shaped, three-headed muscle that runs along the back of the upper arm and helps to extend the forearm. The three heads are the lateral head, the medial head, and the long head. The lateral head (located toward the outer section of the arm) is largely responsible for creating the horseshoe-shape appearance of the muscle. The medial head is located toward the middle of the tricep muscle (where the curve of the muscle group peaks) and the long head (the largest of the three heads) is on the side opposite the lateral head.

The main function of the triceps is to extend the elbow, thus straightening the arm. Unlike men, we tend to carry fat around the triceps, so flabby arms is a common complaint among women young and old. Flabby arms occur through lack of exercise and as a natural part of the aging process. Over time, the tricep muscle loses its shape and firmness, causing the skin to sag. This is why strength training is so important: through regular weight-bearing exercises, your triceps will again become aesthetically pleasing to the eye, and you'll be able to wear your sleeveless tops and strapless dresses with confidence.

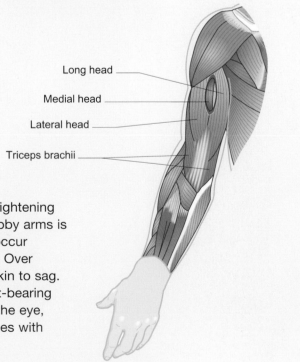

Long head

Medial head

Lateral head

Triceps brachii

cable machine push downs

This is a very good all-around exercise that is most effective for toning and shaping your upper-arm triceps muscles. The best way to visualize this movement is to think of it as the opposite of the standing barbell curl.

level: beginner
main muscles worked: triceps
secondary muscles worked: forearms
equipment used: cable machine
type of exercise: isolation

❶ Take a step back from the cable machine and stand tall with your back straight and your feet hip width apart, toes slightly turned out to help you balance. Hold the bar up near your shoulders using an overhand thumbless grip (palms toward the floor, thumbs over the bar). Keep your elbows tucked in to your sides throughout.

❷ Slowly lower the weight down toward your thighs.

❸ Keep lowering until your arms are extended, with a slight bend at the elbows. Hold the bar down at your thighs for a count of one, then slowly release back up to the starting position. Repeat.

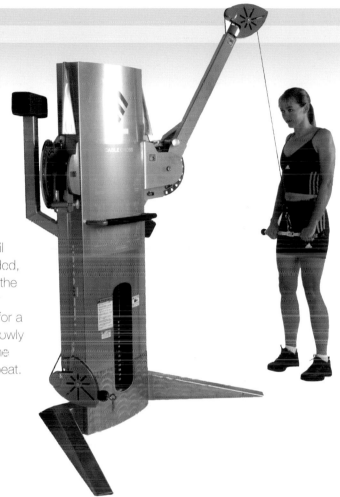

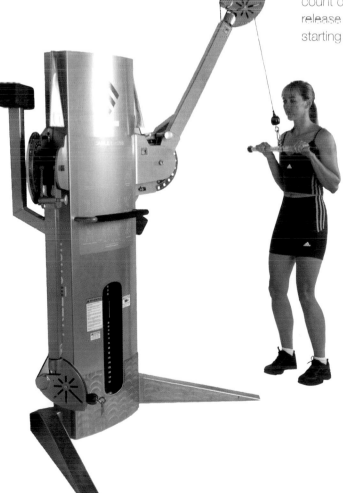

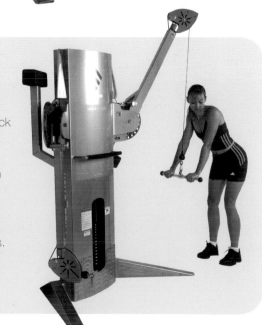

CAUTION
Avoid leaning too far forward or rounding your back over the bar as you perform the exercise; this can place unwanted strain on your lower back and shoulder muscles.

seated machine dips

For those who find it too hard or too uncomfortable to do regular body dips (page 72), this exercise is a great alternative. Once you feel you have built up your strength on this machine, you can go on to master the body dips with a bench.

level: beginner
main muscles worked: triceps
secondary muscles worked: shoulders
equipment used: tricep dip machine
type of exercise: size (mass)-building

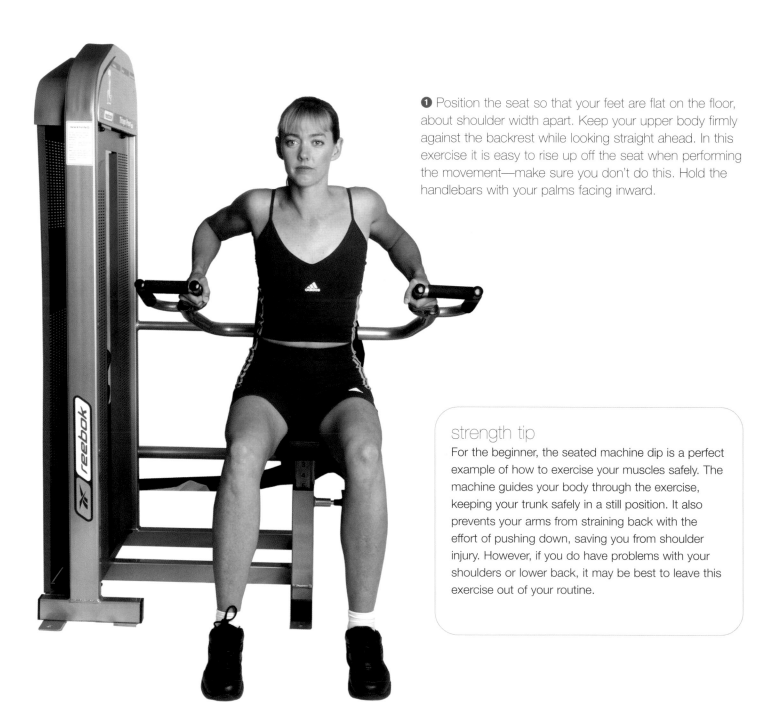

❶ Position the seat so that your feet are flat on the floor, about shoulder width apart. Keep your upper body firmly against the backrest while looking straight ahead. In this exercise it is easy to rise up off the seat when performing the movement—make sure you don't do this. Hold the handlebars with your palms facing inward.

strength tip

For the beginner, the seated machine dip is a perfect example of how to exercise your muscles safely. The machine guides your body through the exercise, keeping your trunk safely in a still position. It also prevents your arms from straining back with the effort of pushing down, saving you from shoulder injury. However, if you do have problems with your shoulders or lower back, it may be best to leave this exercise out of your routine.

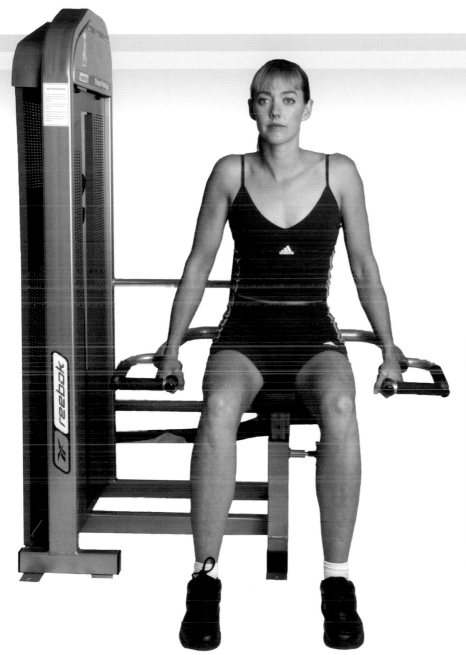

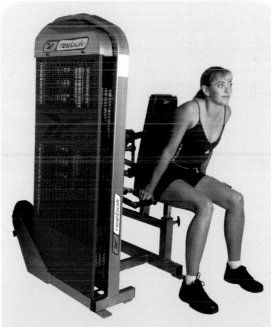

❷ Slowly, in one continuous movement, straighten your arms, stopping just short of lock-out (maintain a slight bend in the elbow). Your elbows should be firmly by your side.

❸ Hold the exercise at the bottom of the movement for a count of one before slowly raising the weight back to starting position. Make sure the weights don't touch the machine plate stack.

CAUTION

Be careful not to hunch your shoulders or lean forward to take the weight (see picture). Always make sure you lift a weight you can manage for at least one or two reps. Don't try to lift too much; you may end up using other muscle groups and injuring yourself in the process.

bench dips

This is another exercise that is excellent for working the backs of the upper arms (triceps). As a beginner, you may start by lifting only your own body weight, but don't be misled into thinking that this is not working you sufficiently. Many people find this exercise to be much harder than it looks!

level: beginner
main muscles worked: triceps
secondary muscles worked: chest, shoulders, forearms
equipment used: bench
type of exercise: size (mass)-building

❶ Position yourself so that your back is facing a bench or chair. Place your feet in front of you, a comfortable distance apart. Your legs should be far enough away from the bench for you to comfortably lower your body so that your arms end up bent a 90-degree angle. Position your hands on the end of the bench right beside your body. Your elbows should point straight back throughout the entire movement to effectively isolate the triceps muscle. Your arms should be extended with a slight bend at the elbow.

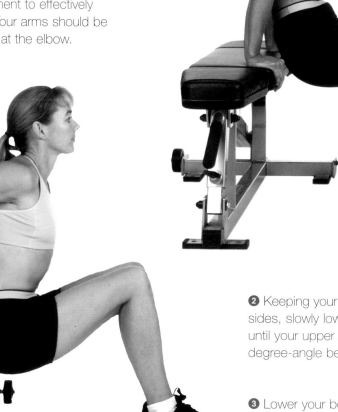

❷ Keeping your elbows as close as possible to your sides, slowly lower your body straight down to the floor until your upper arms are parallel to the floor (with a 90-degree-angle bend at the elbows).

❸ Lower your body, keeping your upper body straight, your hips directly under you, until your elbows are at a 90-degree angle and your legs are at slightly less than 90 degrees. Hold for a count of one, then slowly straighten your arms and return to the starting position.

strength tip

As you get stronger, you will find that lifting your own body weight becomes too easy. You can vary this exercise by raising your legs on another bench and, once you have become more advanced, you can also try placing a weight plate on your thighs.

VARIATIONS

chair dips, dips between two benches, seated machine dips

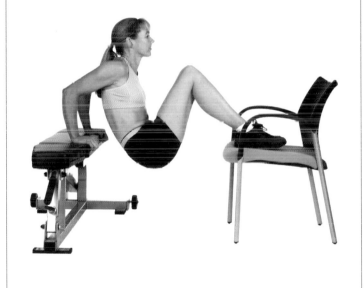

CAUTION

Avoid swaying back as you attempt this exercise. This can put unnecessary strain on the shoulders and prevents you from exercising the triceps efficiently. Your hips should stay as close to the bench as possible throughout.

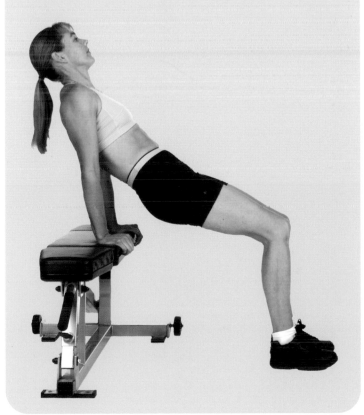

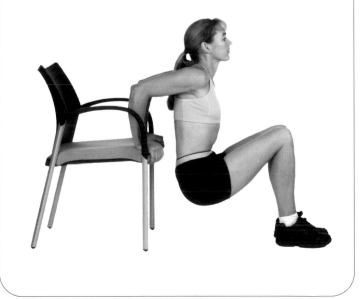

seated two-arm dumbbell overhead extensions

There are many variations on this movement. It can be performed either seated or standing, using a cable machine or with one or two dumbbells, or assisted, using a towel and a person standing behind you holding the towel for resistance.

level: intermediate

main muscles worked: triceps

secondary muscles worked: none

equipment used: bench, dumbbell

type of exercise: isolation exercise

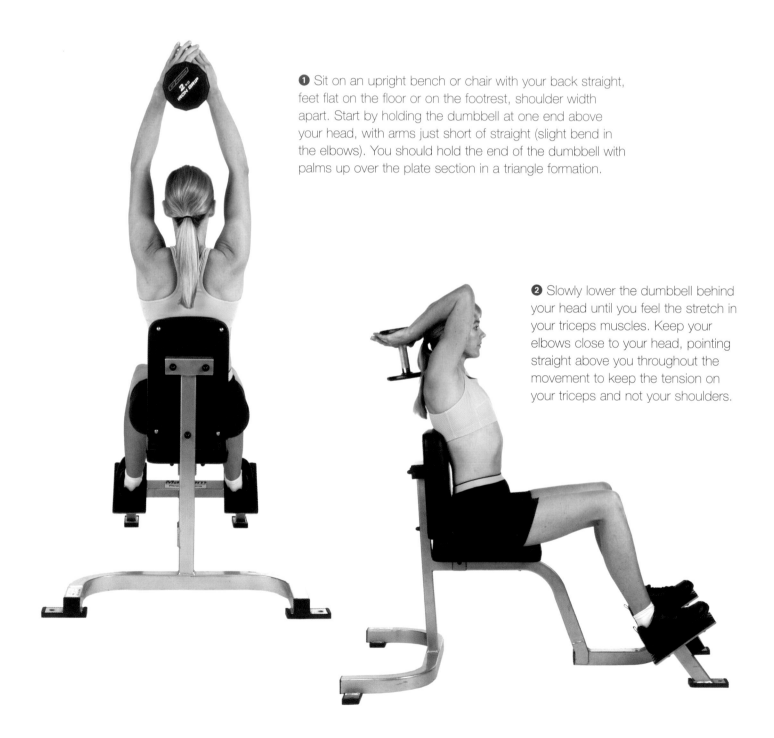

❶ Sit on an upright bench or chair with your back straight, feet flat on the floor or on the footrest, shoulder width apart. Start by holding the dumbbell at one end above your head, with arms just short of straight (slight bend in the elbows). You should hold the end of the dumbbell with palms up over the plate section in a triangle formation.

❷ Slowly lower the dumbbell behind your head until you feel the stretch in your triceps muscles. Keep your elbows close to your head, pointing straight above you throughout the movement to keep the tension on your triceps and not your shoulders.

Always make sure your elbows are pointed up. Don't let them flare out to the sides as this can place stress on them. Make sure you hold the dumbbell with palms under the plate instead of holding it on the side. A firm grip is important so that you don't drop the weight and hurt yourself. If you are concerned about your ability to complete this exercise, have a spotter standing behind you ready to take the weight.

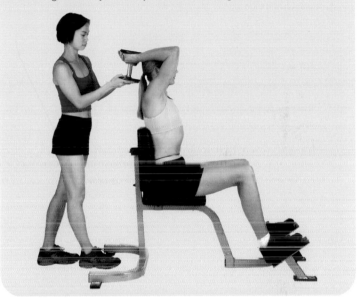

VARIATION

As an easier variation on this exercise, you can train with the end of a towel held in your hands. A spotter stands behind you holding the other end of the towel and pulls against you to provide resistance.

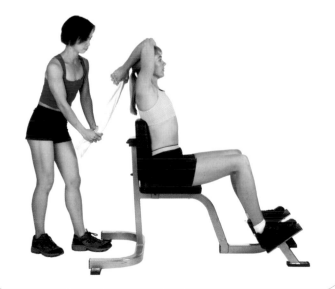

❸ Ideally—depending on how flexible your triceps muscles are and how comfortable the exercise feels to you—at the bottom of the movement your forearms should be resting on your biceps muscles. Hold for a count of one and then slowly raise the dumbbell up to the starting position, following an arc (so you don't bang the back of your head with the weight).

triceps push-ups

Most people hate push-ups. As a teenager, I had to do a hundred push-ups a day in physical education class. I had no idea of the benefit of such a simple exercise.

level: intermediate

main muscles worked: triceps

secondary muscles worked: chest

equipment used: none

type of exercise: size (mass)-building

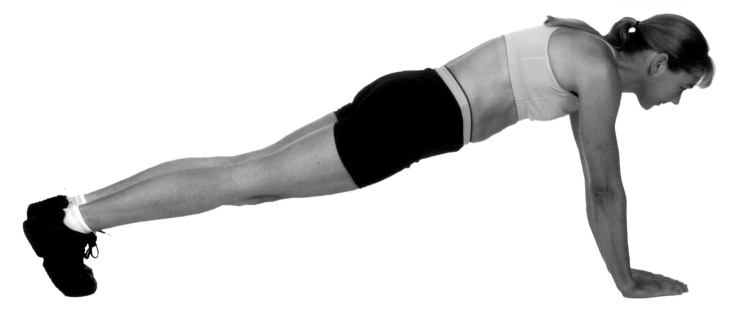

❶ Start with your legs straight (toes on floor; or kneel on the floor if you prefer). Place your hands in front of you, directly under your shoulders, a little less than shoulder width apart. Your body should be in a straight line from your head to your toes. Start with your arms straight and your elbows bent a little.

❷ Keeping your head and neck in line with your body and your eyes focused straight down at the floor, slowly lower yourself, bending your elbows until you are nearly touching the floor.

strength tip

To add variety to your routine, or if you do not have access to any weights, the push-up is a strength exercise that can be performed anywhere. If you are sufficiently strong, keep your legs straight as you lift and lower. If not, position yourself on your hands and knees to perform this exercise.

CAUTION

Avoid arching your back as you lower your body; this places stress on the lower back.

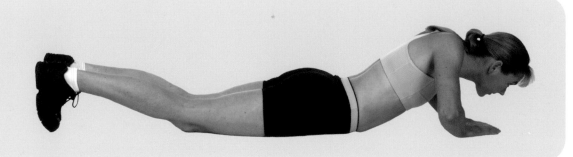

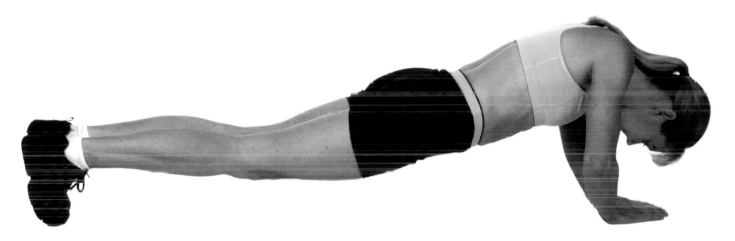

3 Lower yourself as far as you can, keeping your elbows close to your sides. Hold for a count of one, then push your body away from the floor, and raise back up to the starting position.

VARIATIONS

The beginner can perform a variation on this routine from a kneeling position (see below).

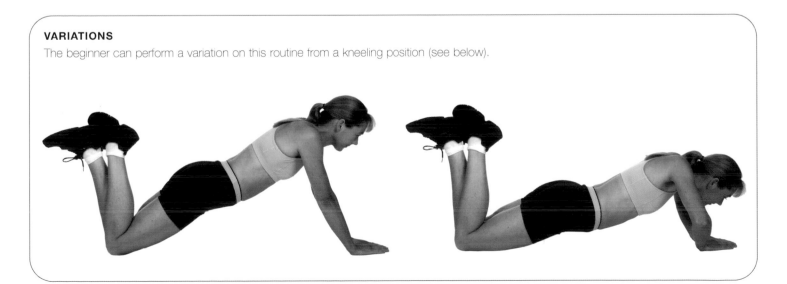

bench dumbbell kickbacks

Although this exercise may appear to be quite simple, it is somewhat difficult to perform because you are unable to look into a mirror to check that you are doing the exercise correctly. You have to trust your judgment and feel whether your body is in the right position.

level: intermediate

main muscles worked: triceps

secondary muscles worked: shoulders, forearms

equipment used: bench, dumbbell

type of exercise: isolation

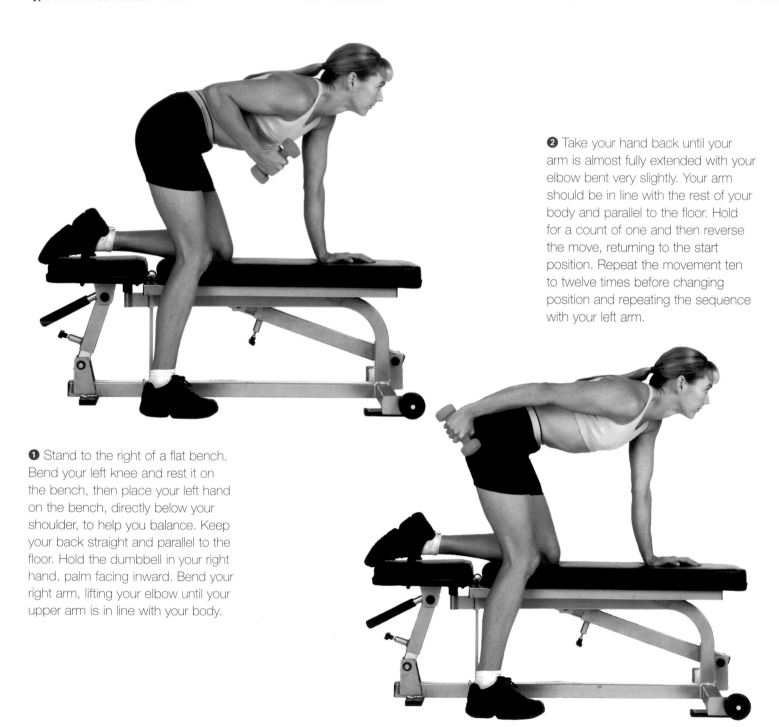

❷ Take your hand back until your arm is almost fully extended with your elbow bent very slightly. Your arm should be in line with the rest of your body and parallel to the floor. Hold for a count of one and then reverse the move, returning to the start position. Repeat the movement ten to twelve times before changing position and repeating the sequence with your left arm.

❶ Stand to the right of a flat bench. Bend your left knee and rest it on the bench, then place your left hand on the bench, directly below your shoulder, to help you balance. Keep your back straight and parallel to the floor. Hold the dumbbell in your right hand, palm facing inward. Bend your right arm, lifting your elbow until your upper arm is in line with your body.

strength tip

This movement is very similar to the cable push downs (page 69). I suggest that you master that exercise before attempting the dumbbell kickbacks. As it would be unwise to look sideways into a mirror to see what you are doing here, I recommend that you have a strength instructor watch over you to make sure that you are performing the exercise correctly.

CAUTION

• Avoid rounding your back, as this places unnecessary stress on your lower back.

• Keep your elbows close to your body throughout the entire movement and avoid letting them flare out to the sides.

• Avoid taking the arm too far back (see below), straining your muscles.

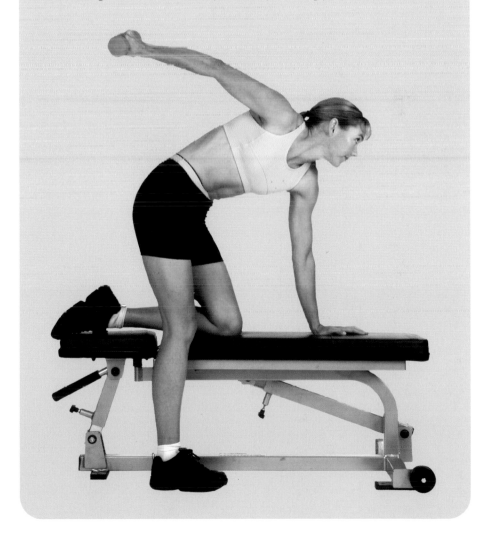

seated one-arm overhead dumbbell extensions

With this exercise you are moving the weight against gravity and placing your triceps under tremendous muscular stress, making this exercise effective in waking your once-dormant muscle and giving tone and shape to your upper arm.

level: intermediate

main muscles worked: triceps

secondary muscle worked: none

equipment used: bench, dumbbell

type of exercise: isolation

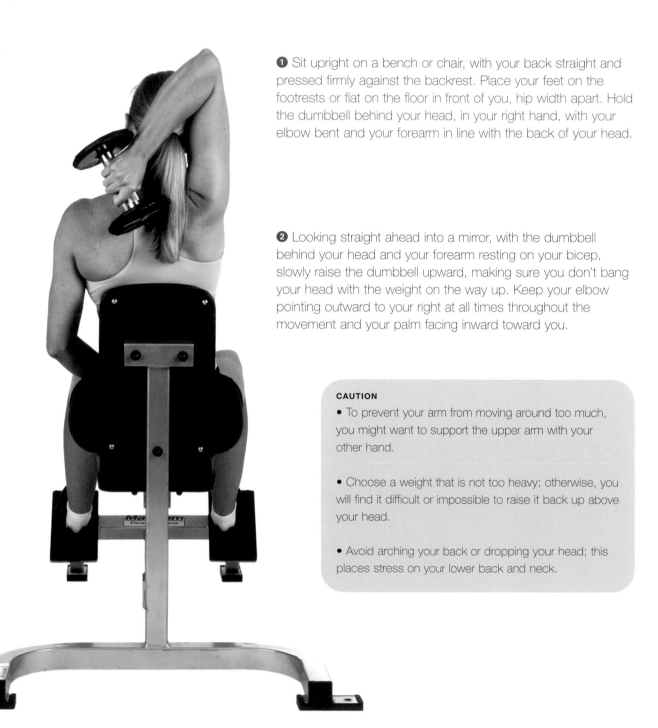

❶ Sit upright on a bench or chair, with your back straight and pressed firmly against the backrest. Place your feet on the footrests or flat on the floor in front of you, hip width apart. Hold the dumbbell behind your head, in your right hand, with your elbow bent and your forearm in line with the back of your head.

❷ Looking straight ahead into a mirror, with the dumbbell behind your head and your forearm resting on your bicep, slowly raise the dumbbell upward, making sure you don't bang your head with the weight on the way up. Keep your elbow pointing outward to your right at all times throughout the movement and your palm facing inward toward you.

CAUTION

• To prevent your arm from moving around too much, you might want to support the upper arm with your other hand.

• Choose a weight that is not too heavy; otherwise, you will find it difficult or impossible to raise it back up above your head.

• Avoid arching your back or dropping your head; this places stress on your lower back and neck.

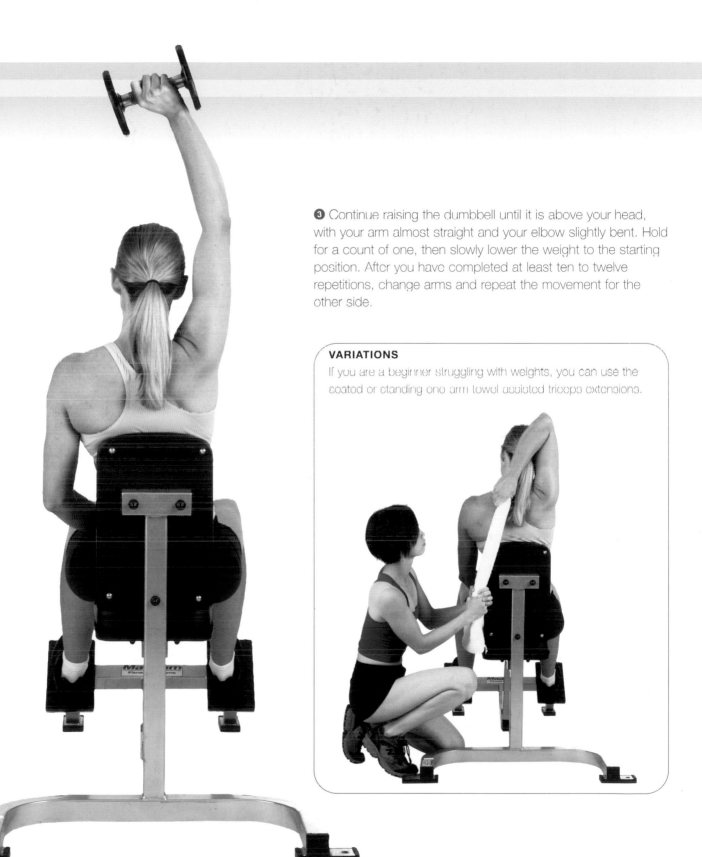

3 Continue raising the dumbbell until it is above your head, with your arm almost straight and your elbow slightly bent. Hold for a count of one, then slowly lower the weight to the starting position. After you have completed at least ten to twelve repetitions, change arms and repeat the movement for the other side.

VARIATIONS

If you are a beginner struggling with weights, you can use the seated or standing one arm towel assisted triceps extensions.

EZ bar close-grip bench presses

Unlike the dumbbells, which allow you move your arms around freely with a more natural movement, the EZ bar keeps your wrists in a fixed position. You can place your hands in the grooved sections for a more natural position that is less stressful on the wrists.

level: intermediate

main muscles worked: triceps

secondary muscles worked: chest, shoulders, forearms

equipment used: bench, EZ bar

type of exercise: size (mass)-building

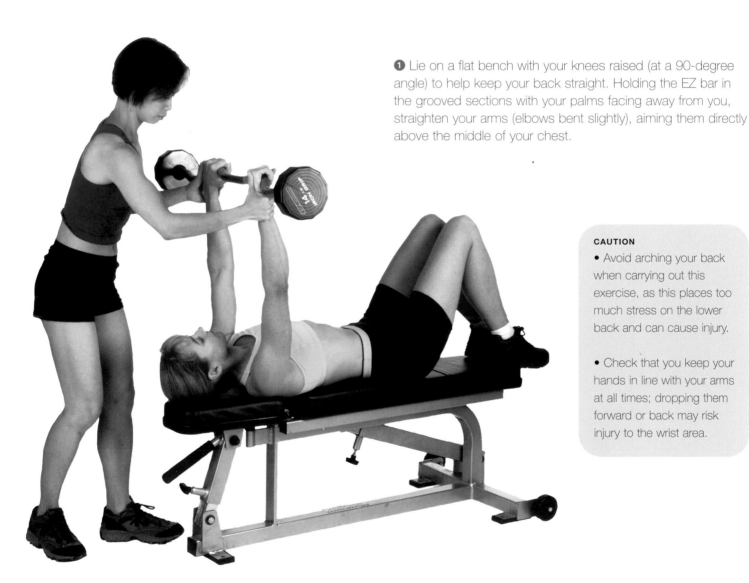

❶ Lie on a flat bench with your knees raised (at a 90-degree angle) to help keep your back straight. Holding the EZ bar in the grooved sections with your palms facing away from you, straighten your arms (elbows bent slightly), aiming them directly above the middle of your chest.

CAUTION

• Avoid arching your back when carrying out this exercise, as this places too much stress on the lower back and can cause injury.

• Check that you keep your hands in line with your arms at all times; dropping them forward or back may risk injury to the wrist area.

strength tip

In any exercise where you are lying on a bench it is important that you have someone like a strength instructor to watch over you. This is partly to make sure that you are doing the exercise correctly and partly as a safety precaution. Although you may start the exercise with a burst of energy, halfway through the routine that energy can quickly disappear, leaving you helpless with a heavy bar across your chest.

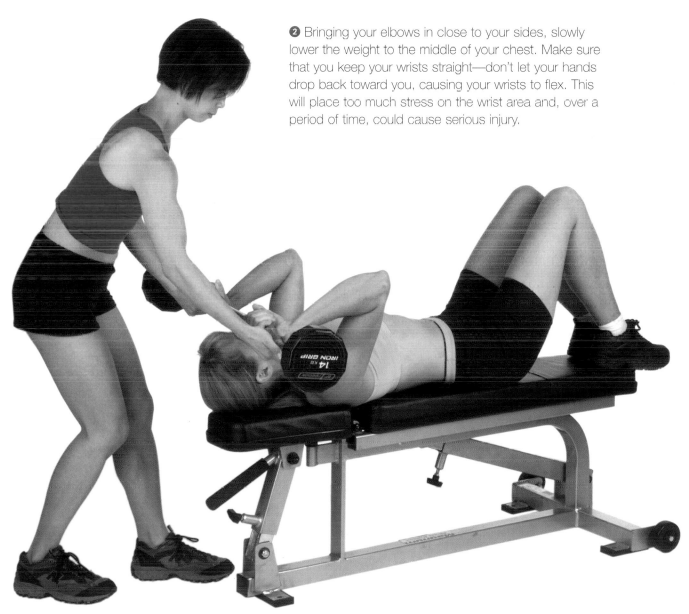

2 Bringing your elbows in close to your sides, slowly lower the weight to the middle of your chest. Make sure that you keep your wrists straight—don't let your hands drop back toward you, causing your wrists to flex. This will place too much stress on the wrist area and, over a period of time, could cause serious injury.

3 With your elbows by your sides and the bar just a few inches above the middle of your chest, palms facing away from you, hold for a count of one, then raise the bar back up to the starting position.

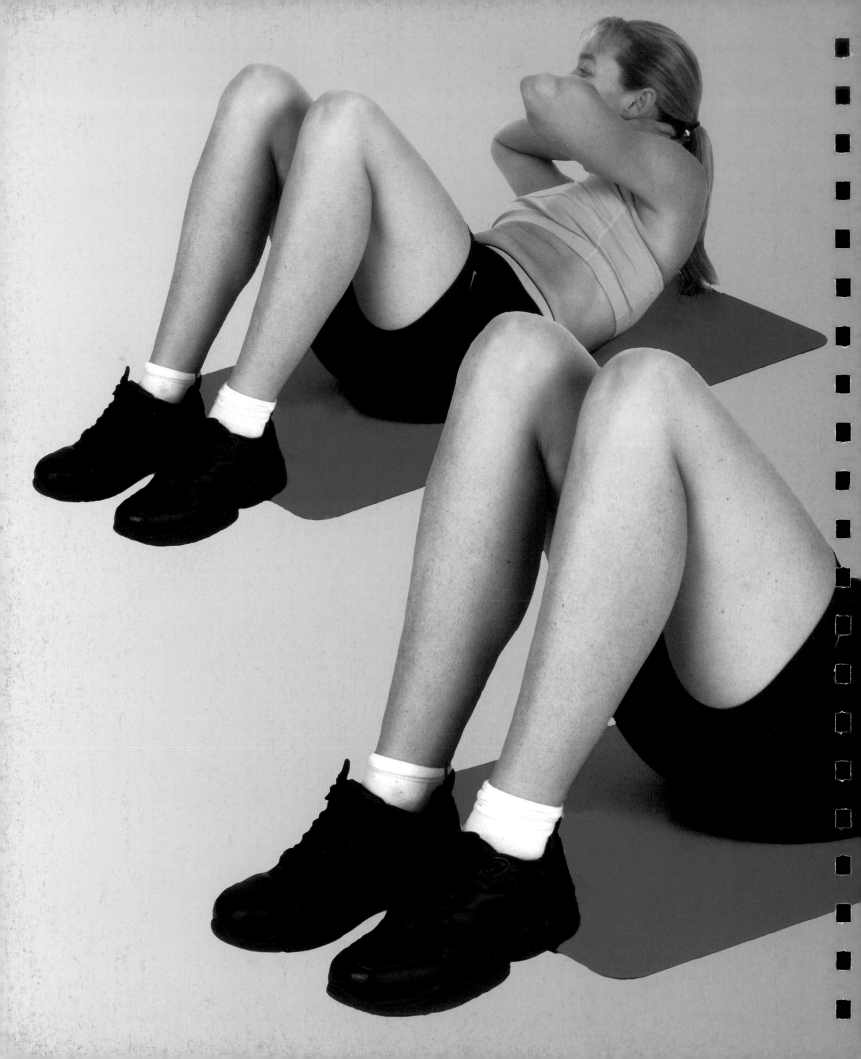

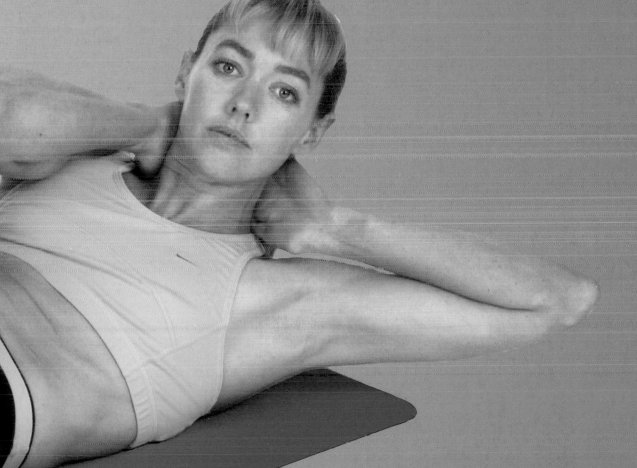

upper body

chest

Also known as: pectoralis major, musculus pectoralis, pectoral muscles, pecs

The chest muscles are fan-shaped and consist of two large muscles, the pectoralis major and pectoralis minor (which sits beneath the pectoralis major). The purpose of these two muscles, when working together, is to bring the arms across your body in a hugging motion and to assist in the movement of the shoulder and upper arm.

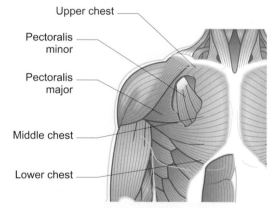

Upper chest

Pectoralis minor

Pectoralis major

Middle chest

Lower chest

There is a common concern that working the chest will decrease or increase the size of a woman's breasts. Breast tissue is comprised of fatty tissue, which is exactly the same as the fat deposits that are located in all other areas of the body. When you train your chest muscles, what you are actually doing is toning the muscle that lies underneath the breast tissue itself.

A reduction in breast size can occur with strength training where there is a combination of intense chest training, a low-calorie diet, and a great deal of aerobic activity. Of course, genetics also have to be taken into account when it comes to breast size and reduction with intense training.

Do not be concerned that if you work your chest muscles you will end up with the chest size of a male bodybuilder. As a female you produce several times less testosterone than a man, which makes it extremely unlikely that you would be able to produce substantial amounts of lean chest muscle in the first place. A woman's chest training very seldom results in her developing a large, muscular chest.

As with exercising any other muscle group, what chest training will do for you is to define, shape, and tone the chest area. This can help to lift your cleavage, which can create the illusion of larger breasts.

In weight training, the chest, as with the shoulders, can be divided into three sections: upper chest, middle-overall chest, and lower chest. It is important to work all three sections to achieve a full, balanced look to the pectoral muscle.

incline barbell bench presses

The upper chest is often a priority for female strength trainers and it may become an important focus of your strength-training routine.

level: beginner
main muscles worked: upper chest
secondary muscles worked: middle and lower chest, triceps, shoulders
equipment used: bench, barbell
type of exercise: size (mass)-building

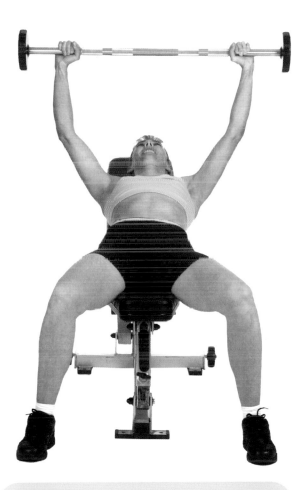

❶ Set the bench backrest to an angle of 45 degrees. Lie back on the bench with your feet firmly on the floor, hip width apart. Place your hands on the bar just slightly wider than shoulder width apart, making sure that your hands are spaced evenly. Hold the bar over your upper chest, with your arms straight out in front of you (and a slight bend in the elbows). Your palms should be facing away from you with your wrists straight.

❷ Keeping your back pressed firmly in contact with the backrest and your shoulders back, inhale and slowly lower the bar. Make sure that your elbows remain directly under your hands as you move (flaring them out to the sides can cause unnecessary strain to the wrists and elbows).

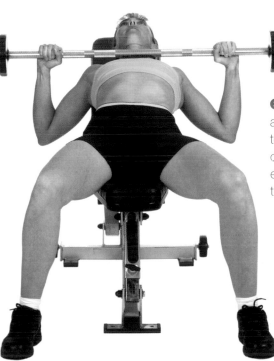

❸ As you lower the bar, allow it to momentarily touch your chest for a count of one, then exhale and raise the bar to the starting position.

CAUTION

• Avoid arching your back as you lower the weight; this will place stress on your lower back.

• Choose a weight that you can manage comfortably—if you select one that is too heavy for you, it could fall and hurt you.

• If you are at all concerned about your ability to lift the weight, make sure you have a spotter standing behind you ready to take the weight out of your hands if necessary.

incline machine press

Here your arms and hands are in a fixed position and your range of movement is limited, too. This is a good alternative to the incline bench press for those who prefer to train alone or feel intimidated at the thought of lifting a weight bar over their head.

level: beginner

main muscles worked: upper chest

secondary muscles worked: middle and lower chest, triceps, shoulders

equipment used: incline press machine

type of exercise: size (mass)-building

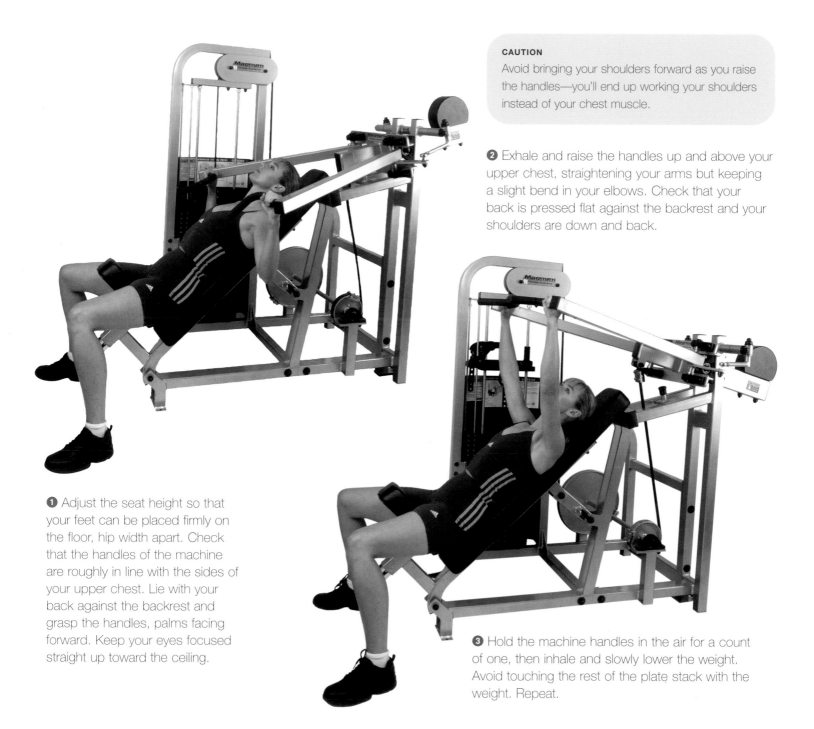

CAUTION
Avoid bringing your shoulders forward as you raise the handles—you'll end up working your shoulders instead of your chest muscle.

❷ Exhale and raise the handles up and above your upper chest, straightening your arms but keeping a slight bend in your elbows. Check that your back is pressed flat against the backrest and your shoulders are down and back.

❶ Adjust the seat height so that your feet can be placed firmly on the floor, hip width apart. Check that the handles of the machine are roughly in line with the sides of your upper chest. Lie with your back against the backrest and grasp the handles, palms facing forward. Keep your eyes focused straight up toward the ceiling.

❸ Hold the machine handles in the air for a count of one, then inhale and slowly lower the weight. Avoid touching the rest of the plate stack with the weight. Repeat.

incline dumbbell presses

This exercise allows your arms freedom of movement; it places them in a more natural position than the barbell or machine presses, where your arms and hands are fixed in place.

level: beginner

main muscles worked: upper chest

secondary muscles worked: middle and lower chest, triceps, shoulders, upper back

equipment used: incline bench, dumbbells

type of exercise: size (mass)-building

❶ Position the bench to a 45-degree angle. Lie with your back firmly against the backrest, feet on the floor, hip width apart. Start with the dumbbells to the sides of your chest, palms facing forward, elbows to your sides.

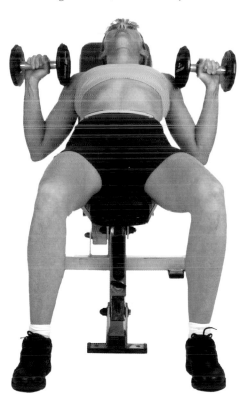

❷ Stick your chest out, keeping your shoulders back. Slowly exhale and raise the dumbbells above your head, straightening your arms, but keeping a slight bend in your elbows at the end of the movement. You may find that you are moving the dumbbells around quite a lot at first and unable to keep them still. If there is someone who can assist you, ask them to lightly hold the dumbbells as you perform the exercise. Once your chest muscle and surrounding muscles, such as your shoulders and triceps, become stronger, you will find it much easier to keep the weight still.

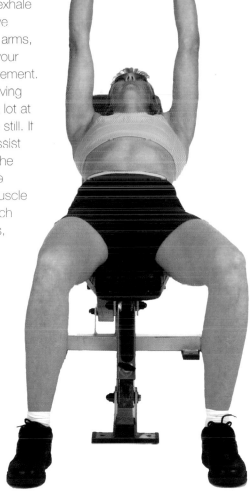

strength tip

Using dumbbells allows you a greater range of movement and consequently works your upper chest to a greater degree than the machine and barbell press versions of this exercise, since the dumbbells can be lowered to the sides of your chest rather than remaining above it. You might wish to position yourself for the exercise and then have someone else hand you the dumbbells. If you are strong and competent enough, you can place the dumbbells on your thighs at the start of the exercise and lift them back as you lie down on the bench.

❸ Raise the dumbbells until they are directly above your upper chest. Hold for a count of one, then slowly inhale and lower them to the starting position.

middle-overall chest

For overall size and shape and a well-balanced chest muscle, exercises done on a flat bench should become a staple in fully developing the pectoral muscle.

Since a woman's physique is somewhat smaller than a man's, I would recommend that you experiment with flat bench barbell presses, seated upright machine presses, and flat bench dumbbell presses until you find an exercise that feels comfortable for you. Using dumbbells while lying on a flat bench may be the easiest, as you can place the weights in a more comfortable position. Dumbbells are superior to barbells in that they allow you a greater range of motion, providing you with the opportunity to work each pectoral muscle separately. However, if possible, once in a while you should also use barbells and machines to supplement your exercise routine and give yourself some variation.

flat bench barbell presses

There is no need to lift huge weights—lift just enough so you feel your muscle working throughout ten to twelve repetitions. Don't forget to ask someone to watch over you as a safety precaution.

level: beginner
main muscles worked: overall chest
secondary muscles worked: triceps, shoulders
equipment used: bench, barbell
type of exercise: size (mass)-building

strength tip

If you asked any strength trainer in the gym to name one chest exercise, they would almost certainly choose the bench press. Why? Because it's one of the most visually impressive exercises for showing off how much you can lift in a single repetition! Don't get me wrong—this is a great exercise; just remember that you're not a power lifter and you don't want to cause yourself a serious injury.

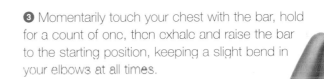

❸ Momentarily touch your chest with the bar, hold for a count of one, then exhale and raise the bar to the starting position, keeping a slight bend in your elbows at all times.

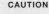

❶ Lie on a flat bench with your feet positioned firmly on top of the bench and your knees bent, to keep your back flat. Place your hands over the bar, at a little more than shoulder width apart, palms facing away from you. Extend your arms (keeping elbows slightly bent) and hold the barbell above your head.

❷ Inhale and slowly lower the bar to the middle of your chest. Stick your chest out and keep your shoulders back throughout this movement.

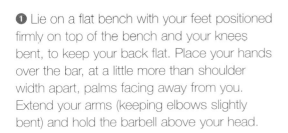

CAUTION

Avoid bouncing the bar off your chest to help get it back to the starting position. If you find you need to do this in order to move the bar, then you are using a weight that is too heavy for you. If you are worried about your ability to lift the weight you have chosen, have a spotter work with you.

flat bench dumbbell presses

In this exercise, it is preferable to have someone to pass you the dumbbells once you are in position on the bench.

level: beginner

main muscles worked: chest

secondary muscles worked: triceps, shoulders

equipment used: bench, dumbbells

type of exercise: size (mass)-building

strength tip

Should you wish to work the sides of the chest independently, the dumbbell press is a good option. As is the case with many people, you may find that one side of the body is stronger than the other. In this case you may want to stick to exercising with dumbbells until the two sides of your body have balanced themselves out and you are ready to progress to barbell or even machine presses.

❶ Lie on a flat bench with your feet positioned firmly on top of the bench and your knees bent, to keep your back flat. With your palms facing away from you, extend your arms and hold the dumbbells straight above the middle of your chest. The dumbbells should be almost touching.

❷ Inhale and slowly lower the dumbbells, keeping them in line with the middle of your chest as you lower them either side of your body. Keep your elbows directly under the dumbbells at all times.

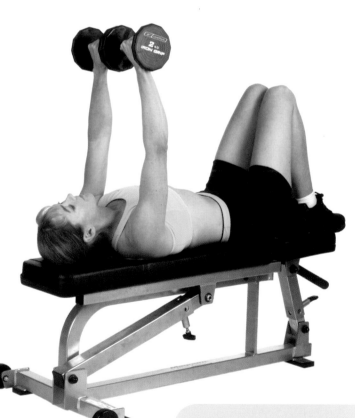

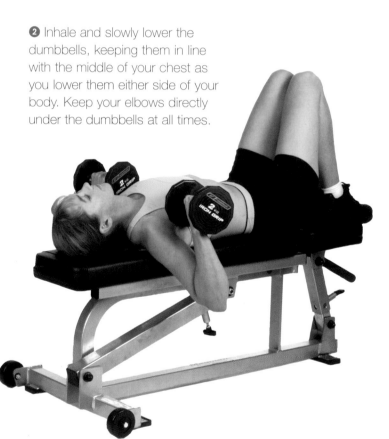

CAUTION

• Keep your head in contact with the bench—lifting it can place a strain on your neck muscles.

• Avoid swinging the dumbbells back toward your head or over your face—they might slip and fall on your head.

❸ As you lower the dumbbells, make sure your chest is sticking out, your shoulders are drawn back, and the dumbbells are positioned directly either side the middle of your chest. Hold for a count of one, then exhale as you raise the dumbbells upward in a triangular movement so that they meet above the middle of your chest.

seated upright machine presses

The seated upright machine press is an excellent alternative for people who do not feel comfortable doing either the barbell or dumbbell press. It can be done without a trainer or spotter to watch over you.

level: beginner

main muscles worked: chest

secondary muscles worked: triceps, shoulders

equipment used: seated upright machine

type of exercise: size (mass)-building

❶ Position the seat so that the machine handles are in line with the center of your chest. Keeping your back and head firmly against the backrest, grasp the machine handles. Your arms should be bent at a 90-degree angle, with your elbows at chest/shoulder level, parallel to the floor.

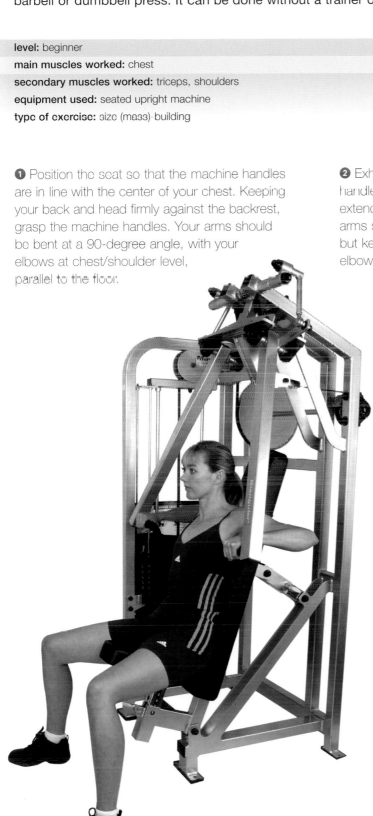

❷ Exhale and push the handles forward, extending your arms straight out but keeping your elbows slightly bent.

❸ Hold for a count of one and inhale, returning the handles to the starting position. Finish with your hands almost in line with the center of your chest.

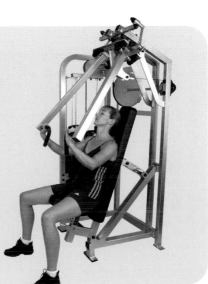

CAUTION

• Make sure that you don't hunch your shoulders; they should remain dropped and against the backrest throughout the entire movement.

• Avoid dropping your arms at any point, as this places stress on your wrists.

floor push-ups

This exercise is a good alternative for those training at home or for those wishing to add variety to their gym-training session. You can perform this exercise either from a kneeling position or with your legs stretched straight out behind you.

level: beginner

main muscles worked: chest

secondary muscles worked: triceps, shoulders

equipment used: none

type of exercise: size (mass)-building

strength tip

If you've built up sufficient strength through regular practice of this exercise, you might like to try a more challenging version—rest your feet on a bench or Swiss ball.

❶ Lie facedown, either with your legs straight (toes on floor) or on your knees. Place your hands on the floor, slightly wider apart than your shoulders, with your arms straight and your elbows slightly bent. Whatever position you choose, your body should be in a straight line from your head to your toes.

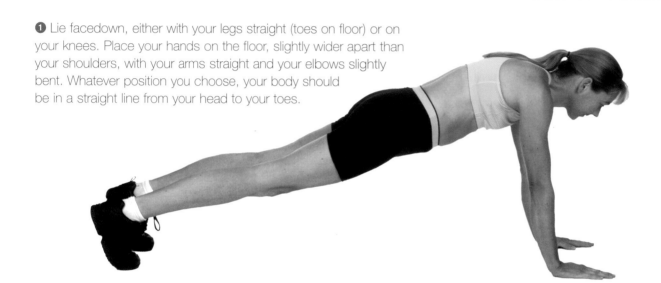

❷ Keeping your head and neck in line with your body, focus your eyes straight down at the floor and slowly lower yourself, bending your elbows until you are nearly touching the floor.

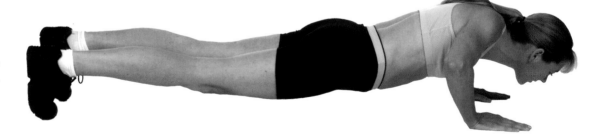

CAUTION

Avoid collapsing at the hips as you lower and raise your body, as this can cause strain to the lower back. If you start to feel any pain or discomfort in your wrists, stop immediately.

❸ As you lower your body, keep your elbows as close as possible into your sides, hold for a count of one, then push your body back up and return to the starting position.

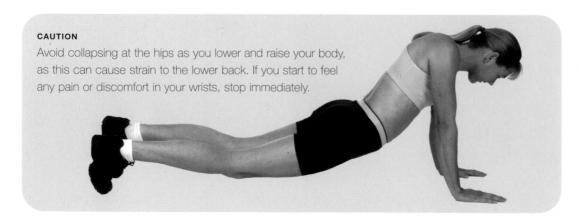

pec deck machine

The development of the inner chest muscle is essential for obtaining overall definition, shape, and separation between the left and right pectoral muscles.

level: intermediate

main muscles worked: overall and inner chest muscle

secondary muscles worked: shoulders

equipment used: pec deck machine

type of exercise: isolation

CAUTION

Avoid rounding your shoulders or craning forward when performing this exercise, as this will cause you to work your shoulder muscles instead of your chest.

❶ Position the seat so that the machine pads are in line with the middle of your chest. Make sure your back and head are pressed firmly against the backrest, feet firmly positioned in the footrest.

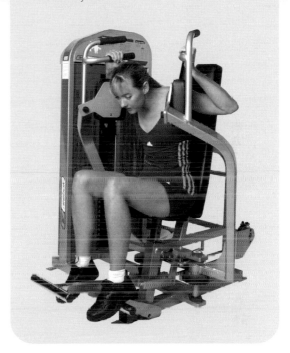

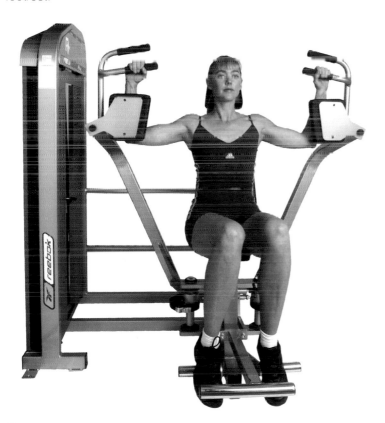

❷ Place your forearms on the pads with your upper arms parallel to the ground and your elbows near shoulder level. Next, exhale, stick your chest out, and slowly press the pads together while squeezing your chest at the same time.

❸ Hold the pads together for a count of one, then inhale and slowly return them to the starting position, making sure that you keep your chest out (letting it drop will take the focus off your chest muscle). As you take the pads back, avoid touching the rest of the plate stack with the weight. Repeat.

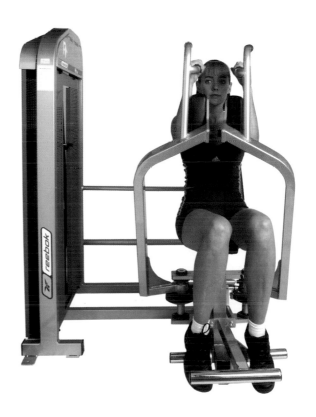

bench decline barbell presses

This exercise rounds out the chest and helps it look fuller, giving it more thickness than the flat or incline movements can do. Although it is primarily used for the lower pectorals, it also works the middle and upper chest.

level: beginner

main muscles worked: lower and outer chest

secondary muscles worked: middle-chest muscles, triceps, shoulders, forearms

equipment used: bench, step platform, barbell

type of exercise: size (mass)-building

❶ Lie on a bench that is raised at the foot with a step platform (see picture). Keeping your arms straight (elbows slightly bent), hold the barbell above the lower part of your chest, with your hands placed slightly more than shoulder width apart.

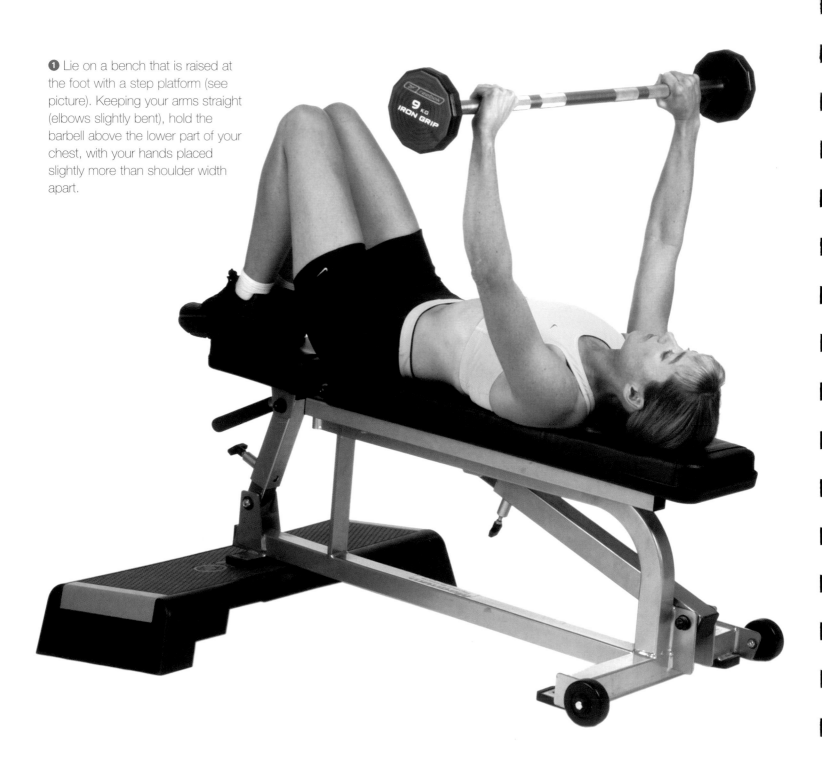

❷ Inhale and slowly lower the bar toward your chest. Keep your head in contact with the bench and avoid arching your back. Make sure your elbows remain directly below your wrists at all times.

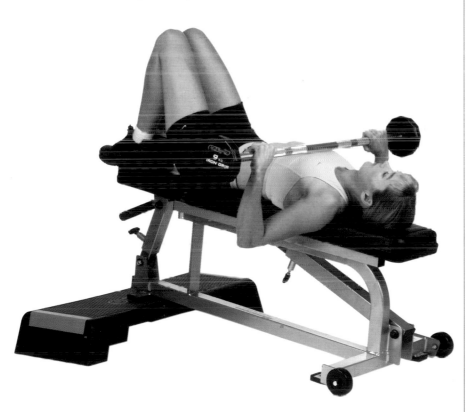

❸ As you lower, momentarily touch your chest with the bar for a count of one, then exhale and press the weight straight up above you to the starting position.

CAUTION
Avoid bouncing the bar off your chest as you raise it—you could injure yourself.

VARIATION
If you are struggling with this exercise at first, make sure you have a spotter working with you.

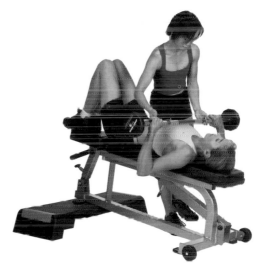

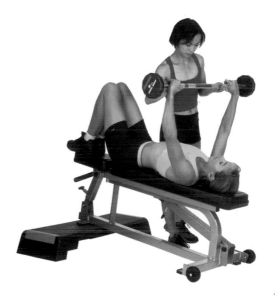

bench decline dumbbell presses

Again, this exercise is a great alternative for those who prefer a more natural range of movement.

level: beginner

main muscles worked: lower and outer chest

secondary muscles worked: triceps, shoulders

equipment used: bench, step platform, dumbbells

type of exercise: size (mass)-building

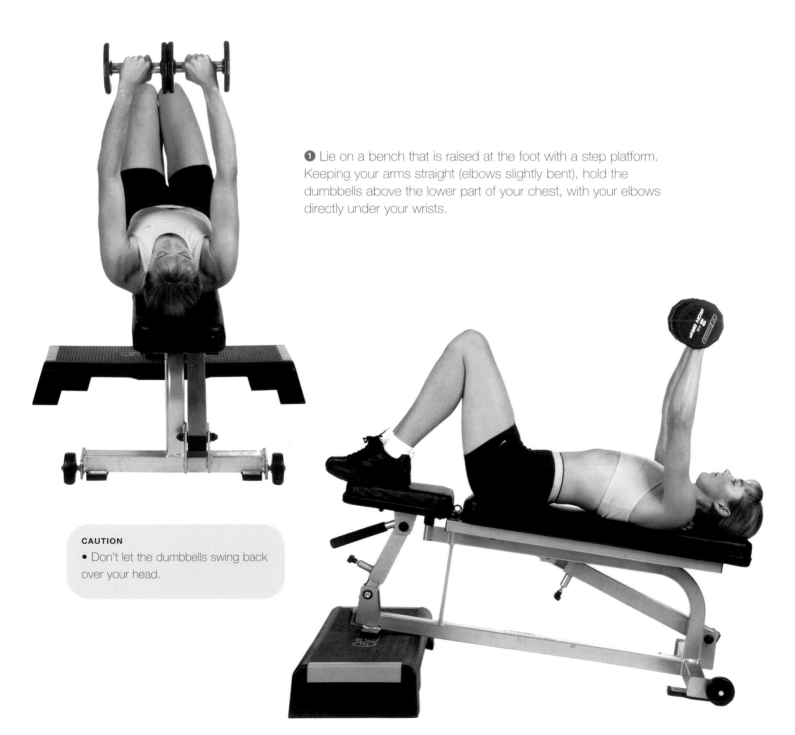

❶ Lie on a bench that is raised at the foot with a step platform. Keeping your arms straight (elbows slightly bent), hold the dumbbells above the lower part of your chest, with your elbows directly under your wrists.

CAUTION

• Don't let the dumbbells swing back over your head.

❷ Inhale and slowly lower the dumbbells down toward the lower part of your chest. If you find that you are unable to control the weights without swinging them back and forward, ask someone to lightly hold them in place as you carry out the move.

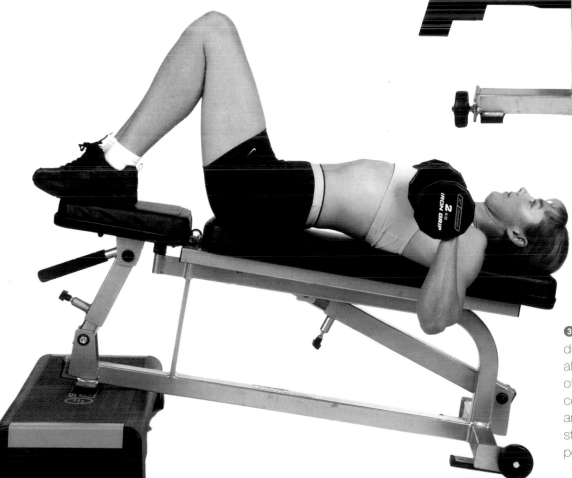

❸ Keep lowering the dumbbells until they are almost in line with the sides of your chest. Hold for a count of one, then exhale and raise the dumbbells straight up to the starting position.

back

Also known as: latissimus dorsi, lats

Everyone seems to admire that image of a wide back tapering down to a narrow waist. The "lats," as they are commonly known in the world of bodybuilding, are the fan-shaped muscles that flare out to either side of the upper torso, creating that impressive V shape to the body. The lats are visible from the back as well as the front of the body, making the training of this muscle group all the more essential.

The lats also cover the lower/middle region of the back, called the erector spinae. People who suffer back pain often have it in this area.

Even if you have a narrow back and wide hips, back training can still help to create the V shape, although, naturally, genetics play a large part in how wide you will be able to develop your back through training.

Time and time again in the gym I encounter frustrated strength trainers who complain of not being able to "feel" the muscles of the back working. Since we tend to use our arms to move or pull a weight toward us, it is very easy for a back exercise to become an arm exercise.

My advice is to try to think of your arms as cables running from the machine or free weights into your back muscles. This image can help you to learn to relax and let go of your arms and concentrate on engaging the back muscles instead. Pulling with your back muscles rather than your arms is easier said than done, but with a little practice you'll get there.

Don't be tempted to give up, even if after a few weeks you still feel that you are training your arms more than your back. Sometimes it takes a while to master the technique of switching off and relaxing all the other muscle groups and working the precise muscle you are trying to focus on. I have been training for more than fifteen years and at times, if I'm not focused and concentrating properly, I still find myself training my arms instead of my back.

Trapezius

Rhomboids

Latissimus dorsi

seated machine rows

This is what I call a "meaty" exercise for overall back development—thickness, depth, and width in the middle of the back muscle.

level: beginner
main muscles worked: middle back
secondary muscles worked: biceps, lower back, lats, forearms
equipment used: seated rows machine
type of exercise: size (mass)-building

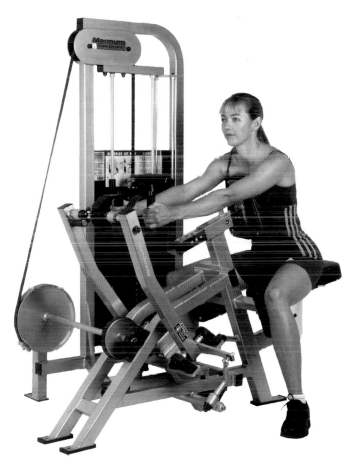

❶ Sit with your feet firmly on the floor. Your chest should be resting against the front pad. Hold the machine handles with your arms stretched out in front (elbows slightly bent) and parallel to the floor.

strength tip

With this exercise it is important to be able to visualize the fan shape of the lats and see them spreading like wings on either side of your back, tapering down to a perfect V. If you find it hard to visualize this, see page 100 or refer to an anatomy book; you might also want to find some photographs of a female bodybuilder's back, so that you can get a sense of how these muscles look when they are clearly defined.

❷ While inhaling, slowly bring the machine handles toward you as far as possible, squeezing your back muscles at the same time and bringing your elbows in to your sides.

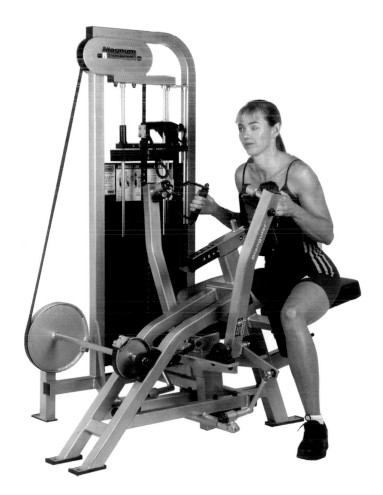

CAUTION

• Make sure that your thumbs are resting on top of the handle, not curled underneath.

• Avoid flaring your elbows out to the side. To fully feel the back muscle working, you need to keep your elbows parallel to the floor and as close to your body as possible.

❸ Hold for a count of one, then exhale and extend your arms forward to the starting position. At the same time, drop your shoulders forward to give your back muscles an extra stretch.

reverse-grip bar cable pull downs

This is one of the easiest pull-down exercises to master. Make sure that you keep your biceps relaxed and try to visualize your arms as cable attachments that connect the machine to your back muscles.

level: beginner

main muscles worked: lats

secondary muscles worked: biceps, forearms, shoulders

equipment used: cable machine with bar

type of exercise: size (mass)-building

❶ Straddle the seat of a high pulley cable machine and grasp the bar with a thumbless grip (with thumbs placed beside the rest of your fingers), palms facing inward and your hands placed shoulder width apart. Holding the bar, sit down, keeping your feet firmly on the floor.

CAUTION

• Avoid leaning back too far when performing the exercise. Your back should remain straight and directly below the cable pulley.

• Make sure that you don't arch your back, which would put strain on the lower back.

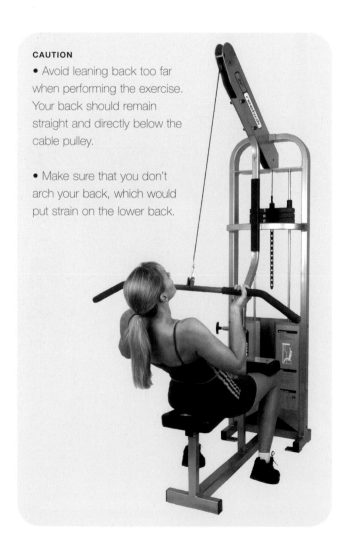

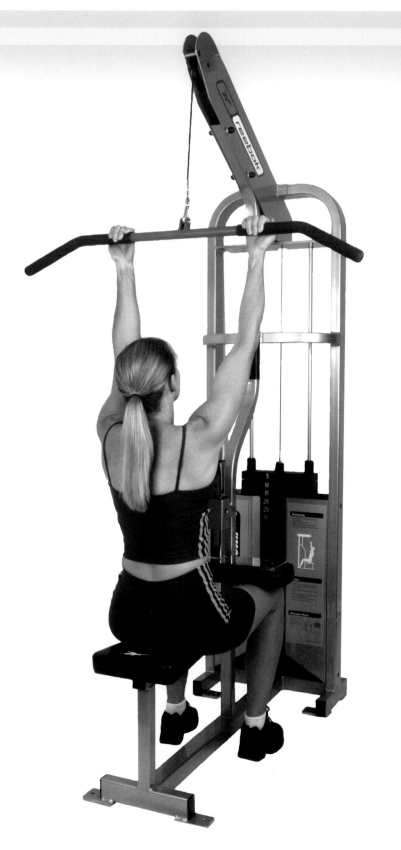

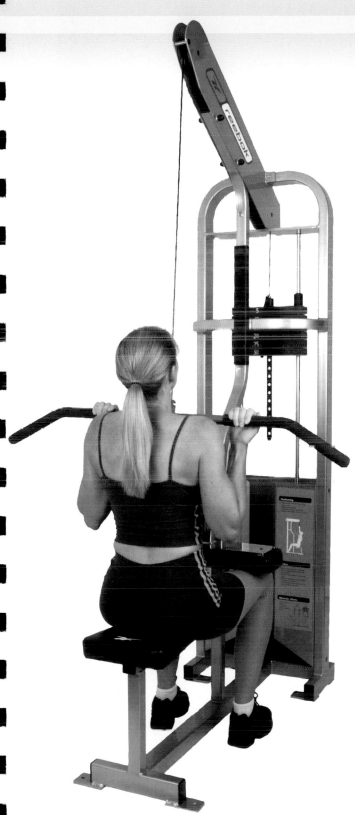

❷ Begin the movement with your arms held straight out (elbows slightly bent) toward the ceiling (see photo page 102). This gives your lats a full stretch before you proceed. Inhale and slowly lower the bar to the top of your chest. Check that your chin is up, your chest is high (it should be sticking out), your back straight, and your elbows are in toward your body when performing the exercise.

❸ Touch your chest momentarily with the bar for a count of one, then exhale and raise the weight straight above you to the starting position.

seated V-bar pull downs

Once you have fully mastered this exercise, you can perform it in a variety of ways—standing or lying down at a 45-degree angle, with a rope attachment or handle attachments.

level: beginner

main muscles worked: lats

secondary muscles worked: biceps, middle back

equipment used: cable machine with V-bar

type of exercise: size (mass)-building

❶ Fix a V-bar attachment to the cable machine. Grasp the V-bar using a thumbless palms-inward grip. Sit down, holding on to the V-bar, with your feet firmly on the floor, hip width apart, and your arms extended straight up, elbows slightly bent.

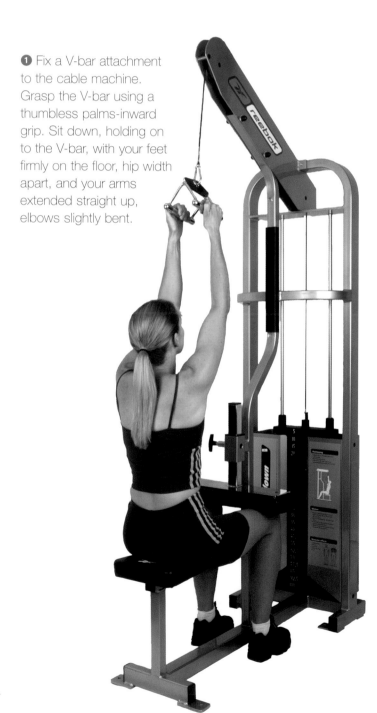

❷ Keep your back straight and your torso vertical and—as for the reverse-grip pull down—inhale as you slowly lower the V-bar to the top of your chest.

CAUTION

• Avoid leaning back too far as you pull down. Your back should remain straight and directly below the cable pulley.

• Make sure that you don't arch your back or hunch over the bar; this could place unnecessary strain on your lower back.

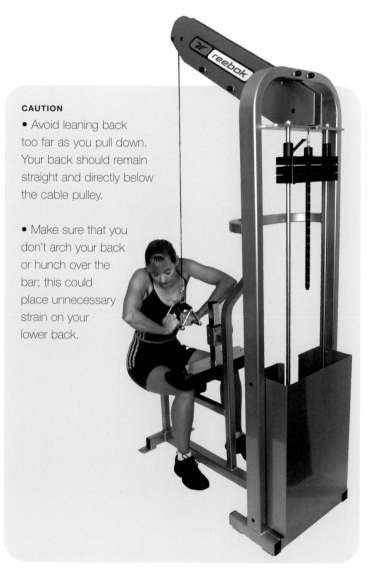

3 Touch your chest momentarily with the V-bar for a count of one, then exhale and raise the weight straight above you to the starting position.

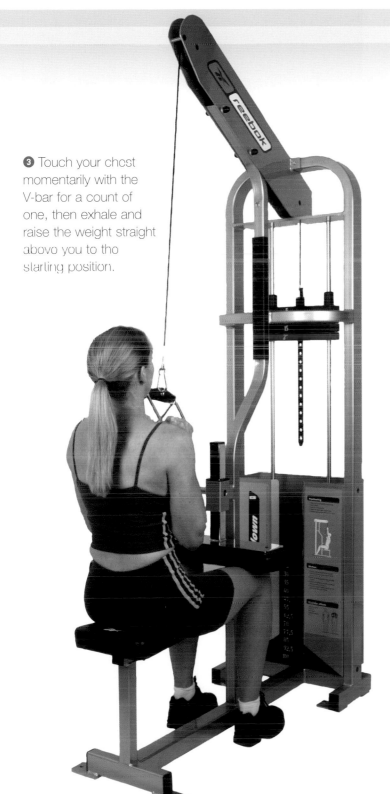

VARIATIONS

You can vary this exercise by standing and resting one foot on the seat or support pad.

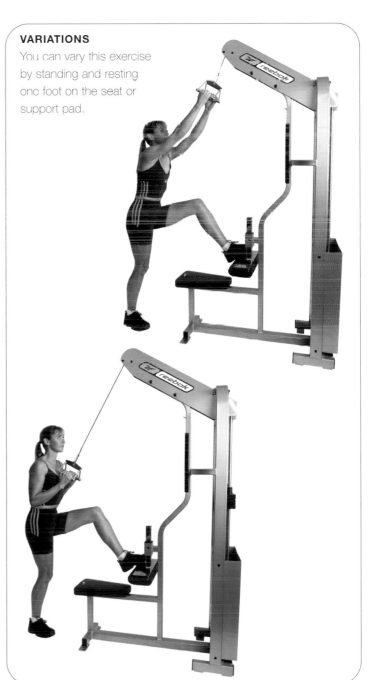

seated overhead machine pull downs

This is an excellent alternative to the bar cable pull downs and a good exercise for those who find that move difficult to manage.

level: beginner

main muscles worked: lats

secondary muscles worked: biceps, middle back

equipment used: overhead pull down machine

type of exercise: size (mass)-building

❶ Sit with your back straight and your feet flat on the floor. Grasp the machine handles above you with a thumbless grip, palms facing forward. Your arms should be straight with elbows slightly bent.

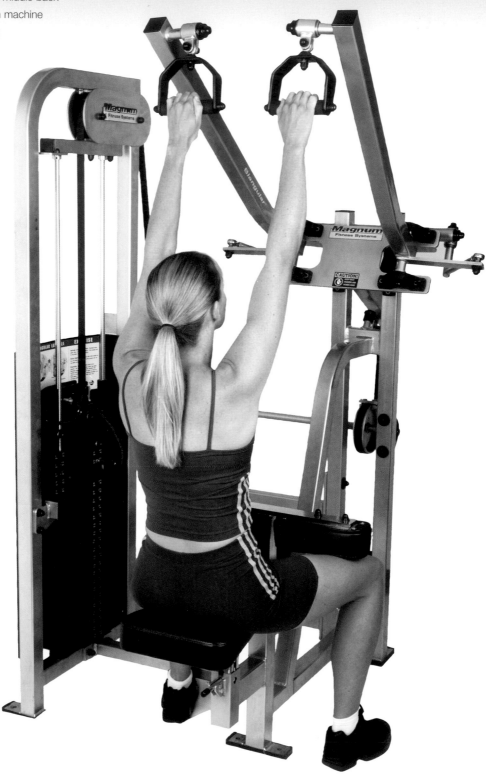

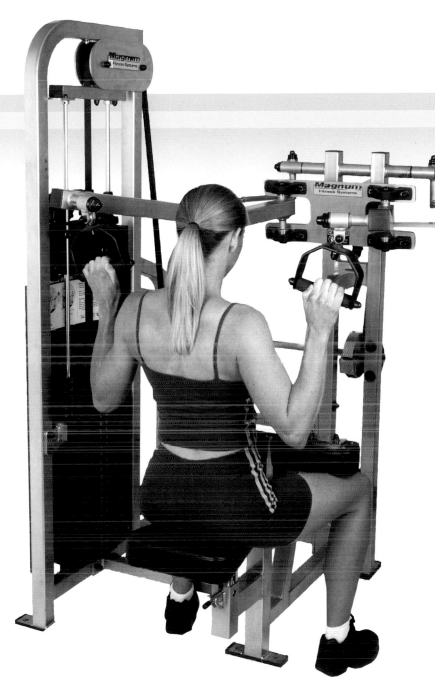

❷ Inhale and lower the machine handles as far as you can, making sure that your elbows remain directly below your wrists at all times.

❸ Pause for a count of one, then exhale and slowly raise the machine handles back to the starting position. As you raise the handles, be sure to maintain a small gap between the weight you are moving and the machine plate stack. This means that you will keep continuous tension on the back muscle during the entire exercise sequence.

CAUTION

• Avoid leaning back too far as you perform this exercise or you risk straining the lower back and will not exercise the relevant muscles correctly.

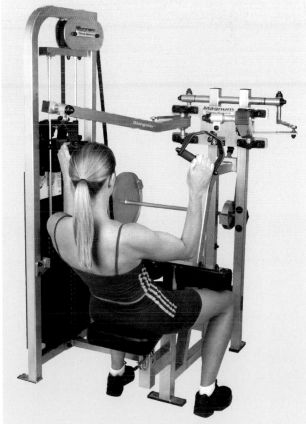

one-arm dumbbell rows

Once you have mastered the dumbbell kickbacks (page 78), you are ready to tackle this exercise. The position of the body is the same, but instead of extending the weight behind you, you drop it down and then raise it up again. Easier said than done, believe me!

level: intermediate

main muscles worked: middle back

secondary muscles worked: biceps, lats

equipment used: bench, dumbbell

type of exercise: size (mass)-building

❶ Stand to the left of a flat bench. Bend your right knee and rest it on the bench, then place your right hand on the bench to help you balance. Keep your back straight and your spine parallel to the floor. Your eyes should look toward the floor. Hold the dumbbell in your left hand, palm facing inward. Keeping your arm close to your body, bend your elbow and lift your arm until it is in an "L" shape with your upper arm parallel to the floor. Continue the movement, taking your forearm up to meet your bicep.

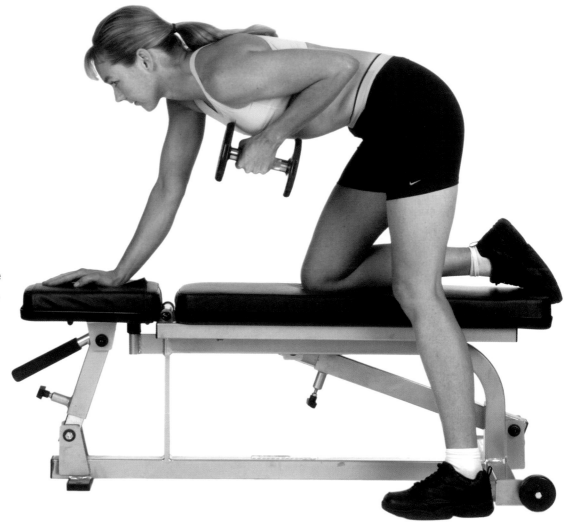

strength tip

To help prevent twisting of the upper torso, you might imagine that there is a pole running through your head and down through your spine and that each end is attached to the walls in front of you and behind you. Or simply concentrate on your body position and focus your eyes straight down to the floor, trying to keep your body as still as possible as you work the arms in isolation.

❷ Keeping your back In position, parallel to the floor, slowly lower the weight toward the floor, dropping your shoulder and extending your arm as you do so.

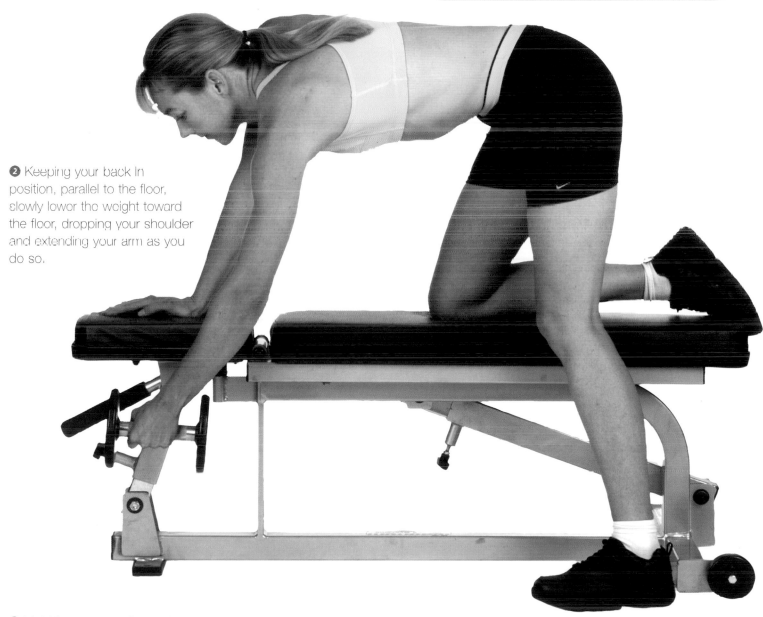

❸ Hold for a count of one, then raise your arm to the starting position. Once you have completed all your repetitions and sets on this side, change position and repeat the sequence for the right arm.

supported machine chin-ups

Conventional hanging chins are very difficult if not impossible for a beginner to perform. The supported machine chin-ups provide you with the opportunity of learning the technique for this exercise, as well as gradually building muscle.

level: intermediate

main muscles worked: lats

secondary muscles worked: biceps, middle back, forearms, shoulders

equipment used: supported chin-up machine

type of exercise: size (mass)-building

strength tip

Since you can use the added resistance of the weight stack to help move your body upward, I would suggest that over time you gradually lower the weight, a little more each time; eventually you will be strong enough to support your own body weight.

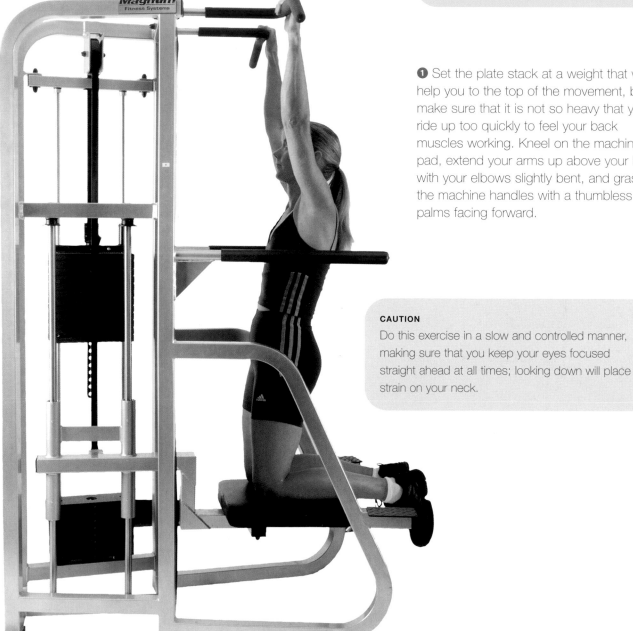

❶ Set the plate stack at a weight that will help you to the top of the movement, but make sure that it is not so heavy that you ride up too quickly to feel your back muscles working. Kneel on the machine pad, extend your arms up above your head with your elbows slightly bent, and grasp the machine handles with a thumbless grip, palms facing forward.

CAUTION

Do this exercise in a slow and controlled manner, making sure that you keep your eyes focused straight ahead at all times; looking down will place strain on your neck.

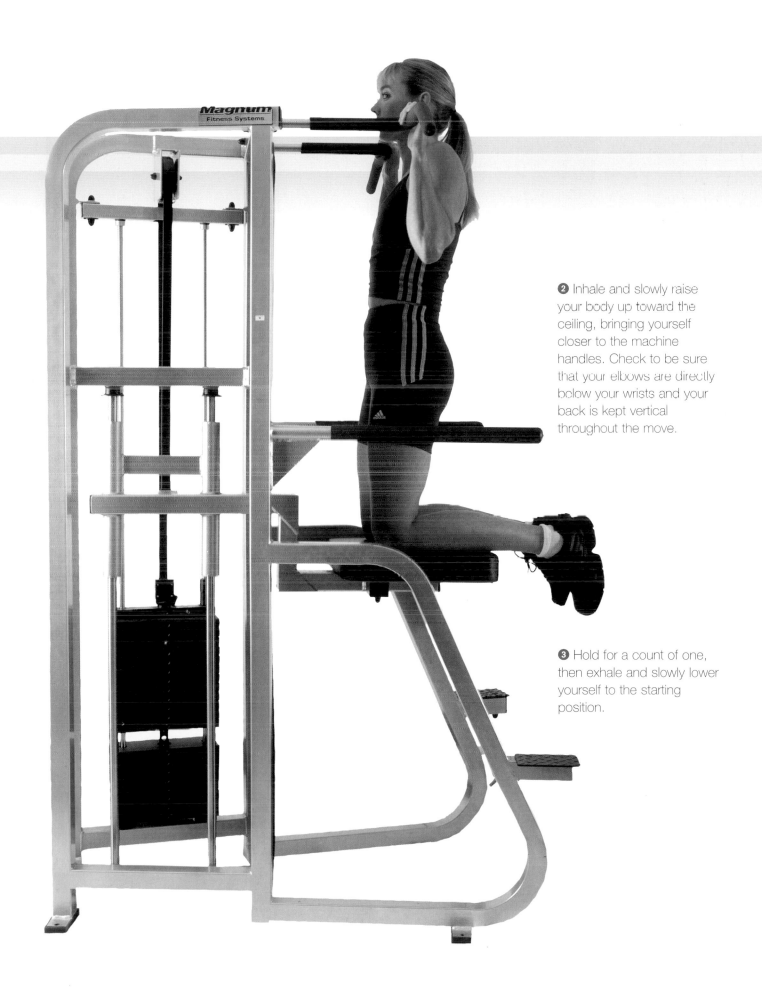

❷ Inhale and slowly raise your body up toward the ceiling, bringing yourself closer to the machine handles. Check to be sure that your elbows are directly below your wrists and your back is kept vertical throughout the move.

❸ Hold for a count of one, then exhale and slowly lower yourself to the starting position.

lower back

Also known as: lumbar spine, lumbar area, erector spinae

Some people consider the erector spinae area to be the root of all evil—for lower back pain, that is. Whether it is because of PMS, poor posture, pregnancy, being too top-heavy (having large breasts), obesity, internal issues like kidney problems, lack of exercise, sitting at a desk all day, weak abdominal muscles, weak lower-back muscles, or back injuries, the lower back is an area in which many of us feel discomfort or pain at one time or another.

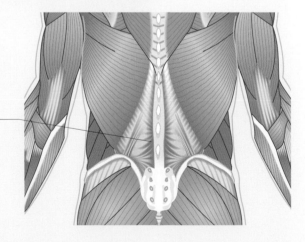

Erector Spinae
(lumbar spine)

To fully understand the importance of training the lower back we need to be aware of its function. The main purposes of the lumbar spine are: to provide structural support for the rest of the body when we are in a standing position, to give movement when we bend forward or back, to allow us to rotate at the waist, and to provide protection for the soft tissues of the nervous system and the spinal cord as well as the adjacent organs like the stomach.

To help minimize the effects of lower-back pain and lessen the chance of injury, it is imperative that you regularly exercise and strengthen your lower back.

floor back extensions

This is a great beginner lower-back exercise that you can do almost anywhere.

level: beginner
main muscles worked: lower back
secondary muscles worked: upper back, hamstrings, glutes (buttocks)
equipment used: mat
type of exercise: size (mass)-building

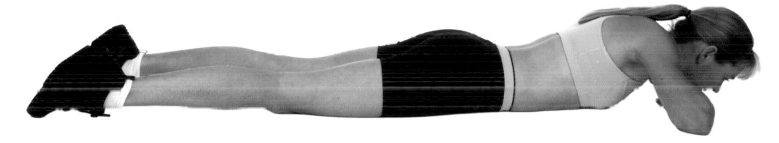

❶ Lie facedown on a mat or soft floor covering with your legs in line with the rest of your body and your feet slightly wider than hip width apart. Place your left arm in front of you, and rest your right forearm on top of your left, as if you were crossing your arms without actually doing the full crossover. Rest your head on your arms.

> **CAUTION**
> Avoid raising your upper body up too far, as this places tremendous pressure on your lower back, which could result in strain or injury.

❷ From this position inhale and slowly raise your upper body and head to an angle of about 45 degrees. This is only a very small movement but is highly effective in isolating and engaging the lower-back muscles.

❸ Hold for a count of one at the top, then exhale and lower your upper body to the starting position.

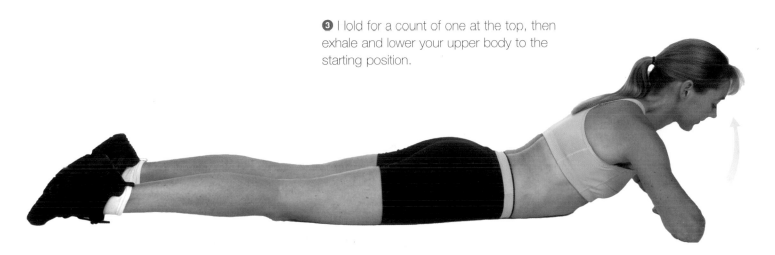

opposite arm and leg back extensions

This is a simple movement but extremely effective for specifically targeting the lower back.

level: beginner

main muscles worked: lower back

secondary muscles worked: upper back, hamstrings, glutes (buttocks)

equipment used: mat

type of exercise: size (mass)-building

strength tip

Make sure that you choose a soft surface such as a carpet, a mattress, or even thick grass to work on. If all you have available is a hard surface, I suggest that you use some sort of exercise mat to place under your stomach for comfort and support.

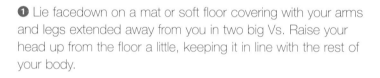

❶ Lie facedown on a mat or soft floor covering with your arms and legs extended away from you in two big Vs. Raise your head up from the floor a little, keeping it in line with the rest of your body.

❷ Using opposite arms and legs as you work, slowly raise your right arm and your left leg a few inches from the floor and extend them away from you, keeping your upper body as still and as close to the floor as possible.

CAUTION

Avoid arching your back or taking your head back as you stretch; this places strain on the neck. Inhale as you lift and stretch and exhale as you release.

❸ Hold at the top for a count of one and then slowly lower to the starting position. Then do the same movement with your left arm and right leg.

upright back-extension machine

Once you have mastered the floor exercises using your own body weight, you will quickly find that added resistance will become necessary to help you further strengthen your lower back. The upright lower-back machine is the perfect piece of equipment for this.

level: beginner

main muscles worked: lower back

secondary muscles worked: upper back, abdominals

equipment used: back-extension machine

type of exercise: size (mass)-building

❶ Adjust the pad that sits against your back; it should be set so that it's firmly between your shoulder blades or slightly under them. Make sure that you fasten the seat strap if there is one, to keep your lower body firmly in place. Choose a weight that is comfortable for you to use; lifting a weight that is too heavy will force you to use other muscle groups (such as your thigh or stomach muscles), and take the focus off the lower back.

> **CAUTION**
> Make sure that your neck is in line with the rest of your body so that you don't strain it.

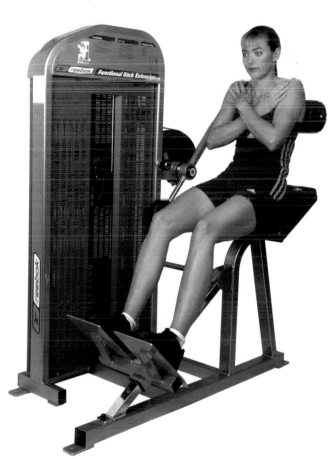

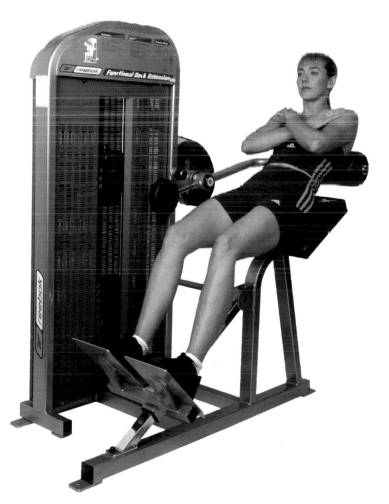

❷ Start in an upright position, cross your arms over your chest, and keep looking straight ahead. Inhale and slowly lower yourself backward to the point where you are nearly parallel to the floor. Avoid arching your back as you lower yourself.

❸ Hold for a count of one, then exhale and slowly raise your body almost to the starting position—avoid coming all the way back to an upright position, as the movement needs to be continuous, with the focus kept on the working muscles (the lower back).

abdominals

Also known as: rectus abdominis, abdomen, abs, midsection, stomach, six-pack

Most women aspire to have that elusive flat stomach. The number-one question on everyone's lips seems to be "How do I achieve a flat tummy?" Well, the main thing to remember is that it's the quality of the exercise and not the quantity that counts. The abdominals are like any other muscle group and, as a general rule, respond to short bursts of exercise with a repetition range of twenty to thirty-five.

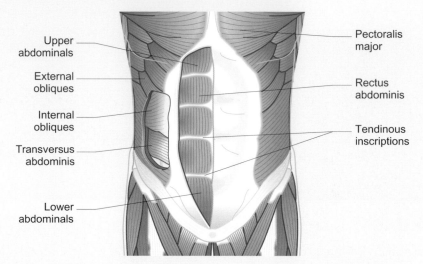

For most of us, the stomach is the first place that we store fat and the last place we lose it from. As with any other part of the body, when you exercise your stomach, what you are actually doing is toning the muscle underneath the fat deposits. Infinite sets of crunches are not the answer to a flat stomach, as you are only toning the muscle and not necessarily burning away the fat around your midsection. The key to a flat, well-shaped stomach is a combination of diet, aerobic training, and specific exercises that work your abdominals from various angles.

As with your shoulders, your stomach isn't just one big muscle—the abdominals are made up of many different sections. Abdominal muscle consists of a thin layer of muscle that starts from the base of the breastbone (sternum) and runs down to the pubic bone area. These muscles include:

Rectus abdominis
This is the muscle in the middle of the stomach that runs the full length of the abdomen. This muscle helps to bend your upper body forward toward your legs; it's also referred to as a "six-pack."

External obliques
These are located to the side of the rectus abdominis. They help twist the upper body from side to side and bend it forward.

Internal obliques
These inner abdominals are deep muscles that lie underneath the rectus abdominis, right next to the external obliques. They perform the same function as the external obliques.

Transversus abdominis
This is a muscle group that lies deep and is located underneath the abdominal wall. The transversus abdominis, along with other muscle groups, helps support the spine.

floor abdominal crunch

When performed slowly using the correct form, the basic floor crunch is one of the most effective exercises for working your stomach muscles. There is no excuse not to have a toned tummy, as this simple exercise can be done anywhere, at any time—in the gym, outside, when traveling, or at home.

level: beginner

main muscles worked: abdominals

secondary muscles worked: lower abdominals and obliques

equipment used: mat

type of exercise: isolation

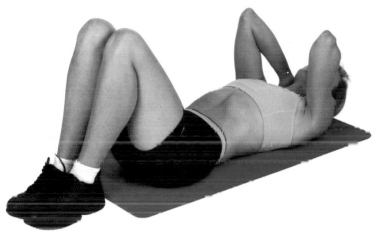

❷ Exhale and slowly curl your upper body up toward your knees, peeling the top of your spine away from the floor. This is a very small movement—only your shoulders and upper back should lift. Make sure your middle and lower back remain in contact with the floor.

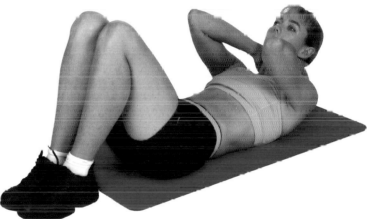

❶ Lie on your back on the floor with an exercise mat or folded blanket underneath you. Bend your knees and place your foot flat on the floor. (Alternatively, you can place your feet on a bench or some other raised surface so that your knees are bent and your shins parallel to the floor.) Either place your hands lightly either side of your head (although if you do, make sure that you don't thrust your head forward as you raise and lower) or cross your hands in front of your chest.

❸ Hold for a count of one, contracting your abdominals, then inhale and slowly lower yourself to the starting position.

VARIATIONS

If you find that your neck starts to feel tired when doing this exercise, place your hands behind your neck to provide some support, but, again, avoid thrusting your head forward as you move, as this can place too much strain on your neck.

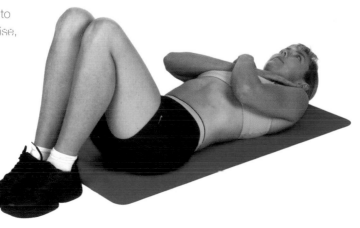

CAUTION

Avoid lifting your whole body off the floor; only a very small movement is required to work the abs. Resist the temptation to pull your neck forward if your hands are placed behind your head—this places unnecessary strain on the neck and spine.

cross-body oblique crunch

This is a basic movement that is highly effective in working the obliques (the muscles to the side of the abdominals).

level: beginner
main muscles worked: obliques, upper abdominals
secondary muscles worked: lower abdominals
equipment used: mat
type of exercise: isolation

❶ The principles of the floor abdominal crunch apply here. Lie on the floor with a mat or blanket underneath you to support your lower back. Either place your feet firmly on the floor (legs bent at about 60 degrees) or place them on a bench so that your shins are parallel to the floor.

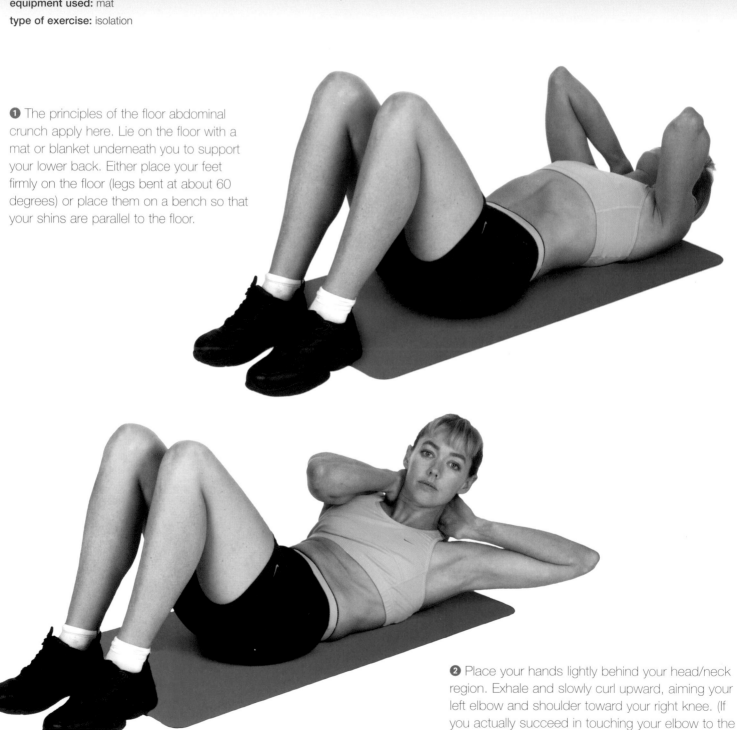

❷ Place your hands lightly behind your head/neck region. Exhale and slowly curl upward, aiming your left elbow and shoulder toward your right knee. (If you actually succeed in touching your elbow to the knee you have come up too far off the floor.)

❸ Hold for a count of one at the top of the movement, then inhale and slowly lower your upper body to the floor. Repeat the sequence, this time directing your right elbow toward your left knee. Continue alternating the arms and legs until you have completed the desired number of repetitions.

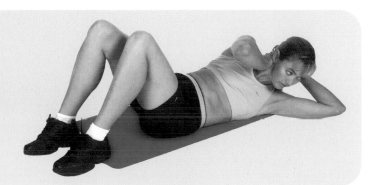

CAUTION
Avoid twisting your body and, as with the floor abdominal crunch, do not lift too much of your spine off the floor as you stretch. Make sure that your lower back remains in contact with the floor at all times.

seated machine abdominal crunch

Once you have mastered the basic floor abdominal crunch, the machine crunch is a valuable alternative. The added resistance overloads the muscles, causing them to work harder, which in turn creates greater tone, definition, and strength in your stomach muscles.

level: beginner

main muscles worked: abdominals

secondary muscles worked: lower abdominals, obliques

equipment used: abdominal machine

type of exercise: isolation

❶ Arrange yourself on the machine so that the front pad is in position over your chest area. To stabilize yourself as you move from an upward to a forward position, either place your hands on the machine handlebars or over the pad.

❷ This movement is similar to that of the floor abdominal crunch, although here it is done in a sitting stance. Once you're in position, exhale and slowly lower your body forward, toward your knees, concentrating on working the abdominals rather than using your lower-back muscles.

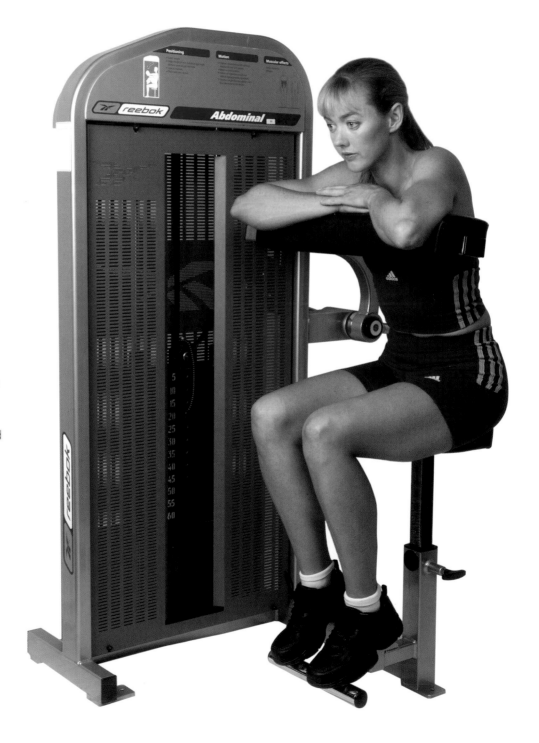

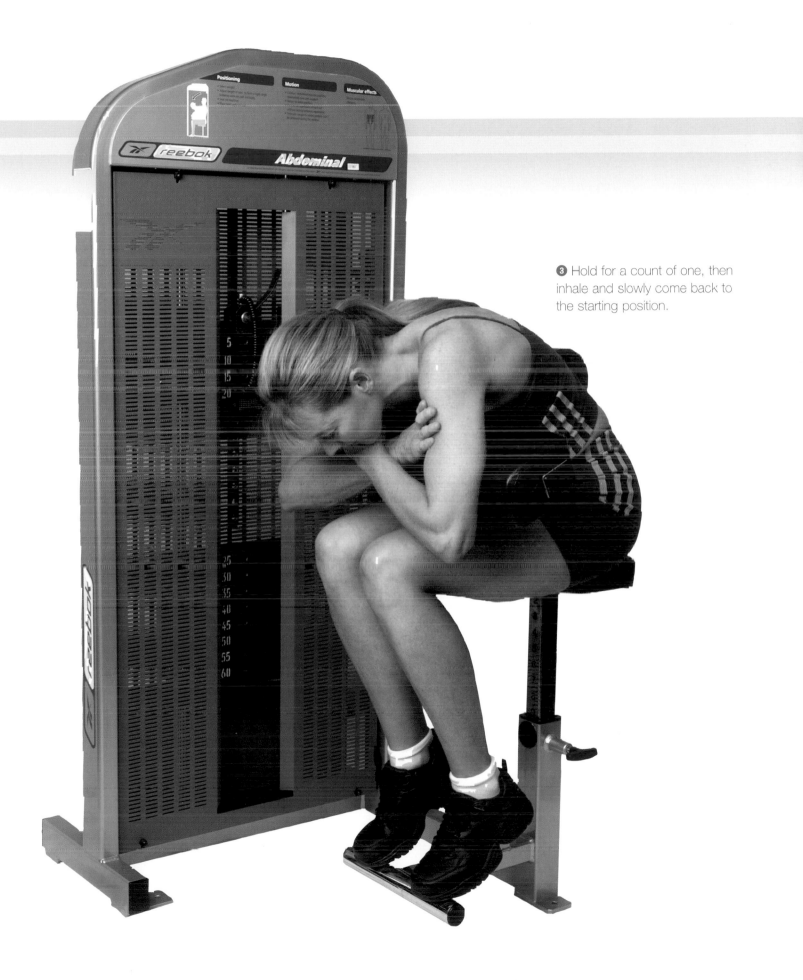

❸ Hold for a count of one, then inhale and slowly come back to the starting position.

reverse crunch

For added resistance, ankle weights can be used. Make sure they are heavy enough for you to feel the extra weight but not so heavy that the movement becomes either too difficult or uncomfortable.

level: beginner

main muscles worked: lower abdominals, hip flexors

secondary muscles worked: upper abdominals, obliques

equipment used: mat

type of exercise: isolation

strength tip

There is controversy about whether it is possible to fully isolate the upper and lower stomach regions through strength-training exercises. It is certainly possible to choose exercises that target one area, but if the movement is done correctly you will really be working the whole abdominal region.

In my opinion, it is best to avoid the whole upper and lower abs debate and consider the abdominals as one whole area. Here variety is the key—if you work your stomach from every different angle, you'll end up exercising all the areas evenly.

❶ Lie on the floor in the same position as for the floor abdominal crunch (page 117) with an exercise mat or folded blanket under your back. Place your hands by your sides and raise your feet off the ground so that your legs are at a 90-degree angle in the air. To find the correct position, imagine that you are sitting on an invisible chair.

❷ From this position, slowly roll your hips off the floor, aiming your knees toward your shoulders. Only a very small movement is required (as with the floor crunch)—it is surprisingly effective for strengthening the lower abdominal region.

❸ Hold for a count of one, then slowly lower your body to the starting position.

CAUTION

Avoid lifting your head off the floor, as this places unwanted stress on your neck muscles. Make sure your upper body remains in contact with the floor at all times throughout the movement.

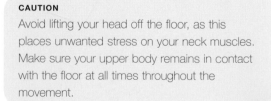

air-bike crunch

There are many variations of the basic crunch and this is one of them. The difference with this movement is that your oblique muscles are isolated far more than with the basic floor crunch.

level: beginner
main muscles worked: obliques, upper abdominals
secondary muscles worked: lower abdominals
equipment used: mat
type of exercise: isolation

❶ The principles of the floor oblique crunch exercises apply here. Lie on the floor with an exercise mat under you, with your hands loosely placed behind your head and neck. Raise your legs in the air so that your thighs are perpendicular to the floor and your knees are at an angle of a little more than 90 degrees with your feet directed upward slightly. Pretend that you are about to ride an imaginary bike.

CAUTION
Make sure you do the same movement with your upper body as you would for the floor oblique crunch. With this exercise it is easy to just flap your elbows from side to side without actually moving your shoulder across your body and working your oblique/upper abdominal muscles. Good form is crucial here.

❷ Curl upward as in an oblique floor crunch. Bring your left elbow toward your right knee as your knee comes toward you in a bicycling motion.

❸ Hold for a count of one, then release and repeat for the right elbow and left knee. Continue using alternating arms and legs until you have completed the desired number of repetitions.

strength tip
For added resistance, you can use ankle weights. Make sure that they are heavy enough for you to feel the extra weight but not so heavy that the movement becomes too difficult.

Swiss-ball crunch

I consider this an intermediate movement and not one for complete novices. It requires a certain level of abdominal strength, stability, and muscle control for you to perform this movement correctly on an exercise ball because the ball can easily move out from under you as you work.

level: intermediate

main muscles worked: abdominals

secondary muscles worked: lower abdominals, obliques

equipment used: Swiss ball

type of exercise: isolation

❶ Sit on a Swiss ball that is the correct size for your height and body weight—you should have a 45-degree bend in your knee joint when sitting on top of the ball. Make sure your feet are firmly on the floor, about hip width apart, to help balance yourself. Place your hands behind or beside your head or, if you are at a more advanced level, crossed in front of your chest.

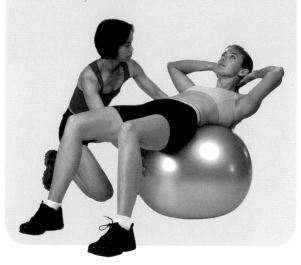

CAUTION

Avoid rushing this exercise—you may lose your balance and fall off the ball (particularly if working with an exercise ball is a new experience for you). If you find you are unable to keep the ball still while performing this movement, ask someone to hold it for you.

❷ Keep your legs at a 90-degree angle and your lower back and buttocks in position on top of the ball, but as far back as possible. Inhale and slowly lower yourself back until your body is parallel to the floor, with your upper body curled over the back of the ball.

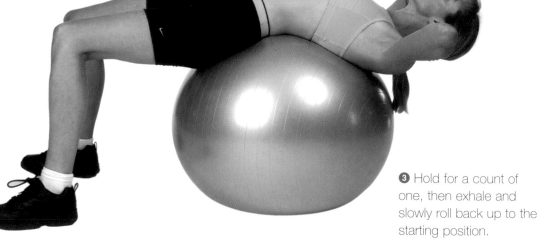

❸ Hold for a count of one, then exhale and slowly roll back up to the starting position.

machine cable rope crunch

As with the seated machine crunch, the cable rope crunch places the abdominal muscles under stress with the added resistance. This extra weight encourages the abdominal muscles to work harder, which improves definition, tone, and shape.

level: intermediate

main muscles worked: upper abdominals

secondary muscles worked: lower abdominals, obliques

equipment used: cable machine and rope handles

type of exercise: isolation

❶ Kneel beneath the cable machine, making sure that the rope handles are directly in front of your forehead. Grasp the rope handles with your hands firmly against the rope ball heads at the base of the handles.

❷ Exhale and crunch your body toward the floor. Your elbows should almost reach your thighs at the end of the movement. If it helps, try imagining that you are curling yourself up into a little ball.

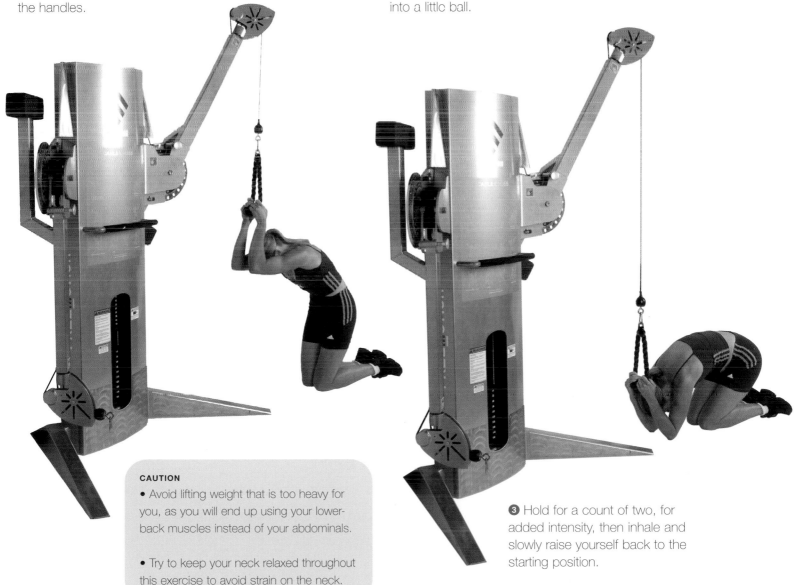

CAUTION
• Avoid lifting weight that is too heavy for you, as you will end up using your lower-back muscles instead of your abdominals.

• Try to keep your neck relaxed throughout this exercise to avoid strain on the neck.

❸ Hold for a count of two, for added intensity, then inhale and slowly raise yourself back to the starting position.

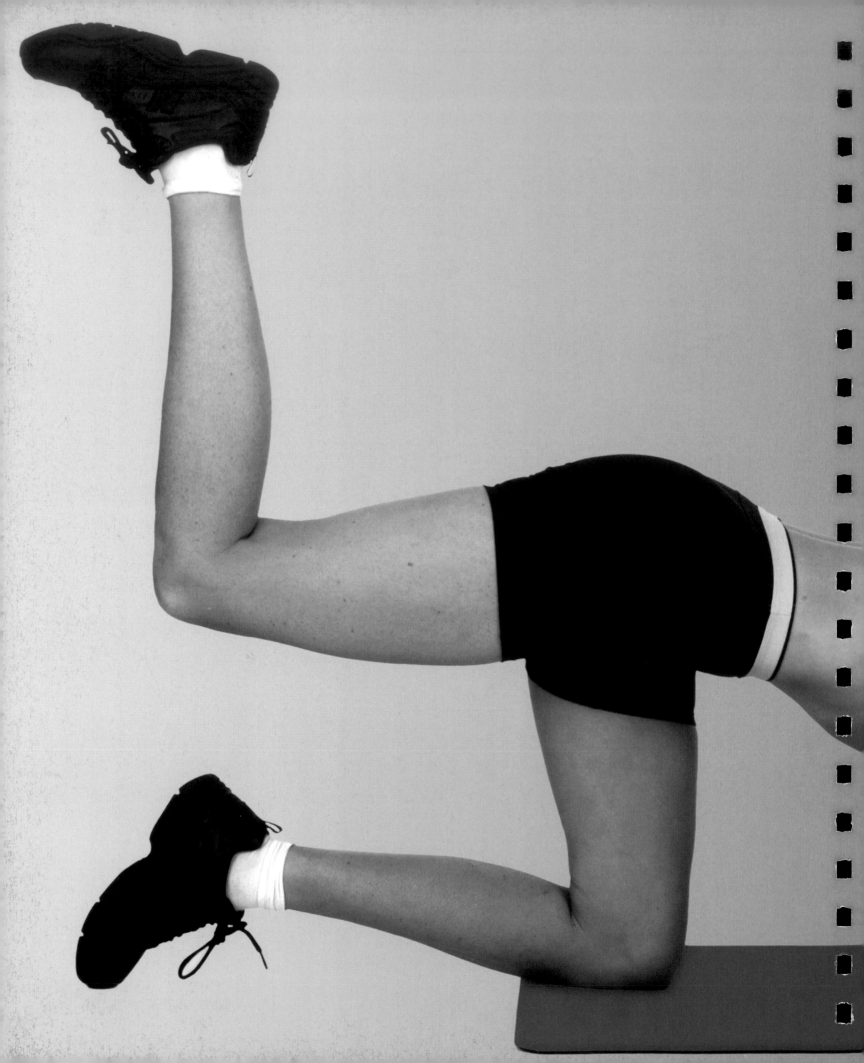

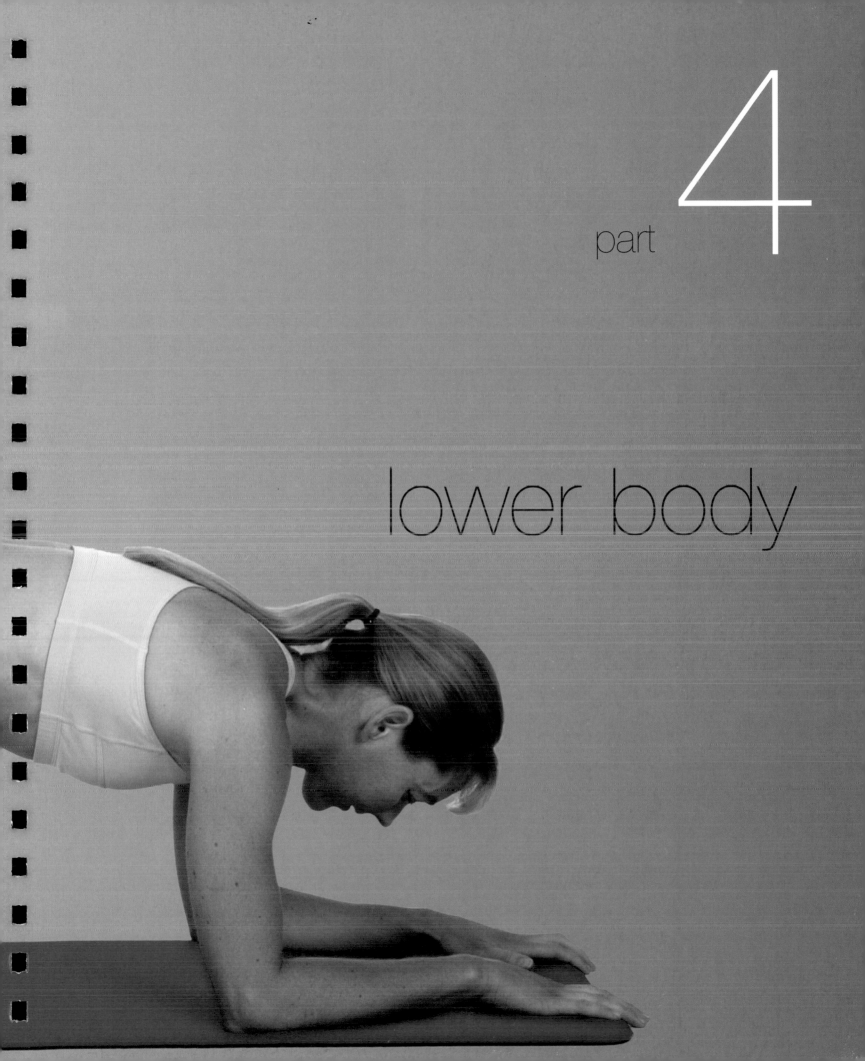

part 4

lower body

quadriceps

Also known as: musculus quadriceps femoris, quads, thighs

Some regular strength training can help give you shapely thighs. The thighs form the main part of the lower body and each thigh is not just one muscle but actually four muscle groups in one. The term "quadriceps" technically refers to any four-headed muscle group such as this.

The four muscles of the thigh are: the rectus femoris, the vastus lateralis, the vastus medialis, and the vastus intermedius. The main function of the thigh or quadriceps muscle is to extend your lower leg forward, as in running or walking. For a leaner, more slender, defined, and toned look to the thigh, it is important to do a variety of different leg exercises that work all the different parts of the thigh muscle.

Weak thigh muscles can be a contributing factor to knee pain. Strengthening the quad muscles that surround and attach to the knee joint will help keep your knees healthy and strong. It will also help protect your knees against such conditions as osteoarthritis. If you already suffer from arthritic knees, strength training can help protect the joint and delay the continuing progression of the disease.

Think of your body like a car. For a car to run smoothly, every part of it has to be in working order and checked and serviced every so often. Your body requires the same treatment. You cannot isolate any one muscle without compromising another, because everything is connected to everything else. The same principle applies if you have an injury. For example, if you sprain your ankle on your right side, you will almost certainly compensate by placing extra weight on your left side in order to take the pressure off the injured right ankle, causing strain and possibly injury to that side, too.

If you suffer from any form of arthritis of the knee, malaligned knees (knees that do not line up correctly with the rest of the body), or lax knees (knees that are loose), it is important that you consult your doctor before starting a strength-training routine.

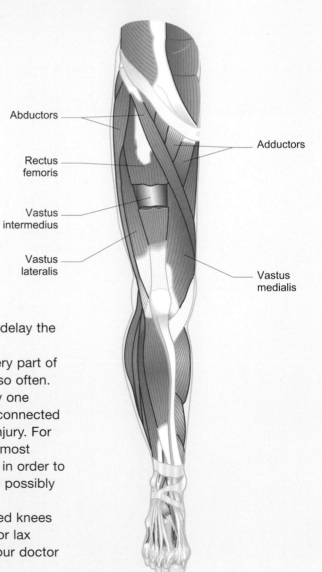

Abductors

Adductors

Rectus femoris

Vastus intermedius

Vastus lateralis

Vastus medialis

seated machine leg presses

If you are looking to increase the overall size of your thigh muscles or add slabs of hard-earned lean muscle, the leg press is the perfect machine for you. If you have very slim legs that are lacking in muscle shape, I suggest you focus a great deal of attention on this exercise.

level: beginner

main muscles worked: quadriceps

secondary muscles worked: glutes, hamstrings, calves

equipment used: leg-press machine

type of exercise: size (mass)-building

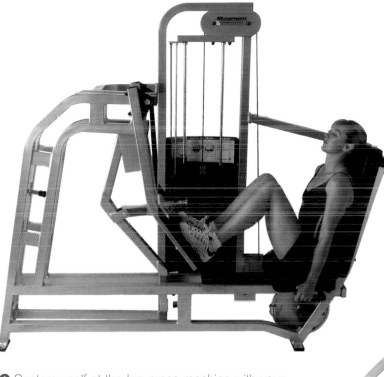

❷ Slowly extend and straighten your legs in front of you, pushing the weight away from your body. Avoid lifting your head or back away from the backrest as this could place unnecessary strain on your neck and lower back. If you find that you cannot perform this exercise without this happening then the weight is too heavy for you at this stage. Choose a weight that allows you to feel your thigh muscles working but is not so heavy that you struggle with the exercise.

❶ Seat yourself at the leg-press machine with your back and head resting firmly against the backrest throughout the entire movement. Place your feet approximately hip width apart in the middle of the machine platform, with your toes slightly turned outward. You should start with your knees at an angle of roughly 90 degrees—or whatever feels most comfortable for you. Your thighs should be a few inches away from your upper body at the starting point.

❸ Your legs should be slightly bent at all times. If you straighten them completely as you extend your legs away from you, you will be placing unnecessary pressure on the knee joint, which could cause strain or injury to the knee area.

seated machine leg extensions

This is a fantastic isolation exercise that solely works the thigh muscles, particularly the lower part of the thigh near the knee joint. This exercise can also be done as a single-leg extension.

level: beginner

main muscles worked: quadriceps, hip flexors

secondary muscles worked: none

equipment used: leg-extension machine

type of exercise: isolation

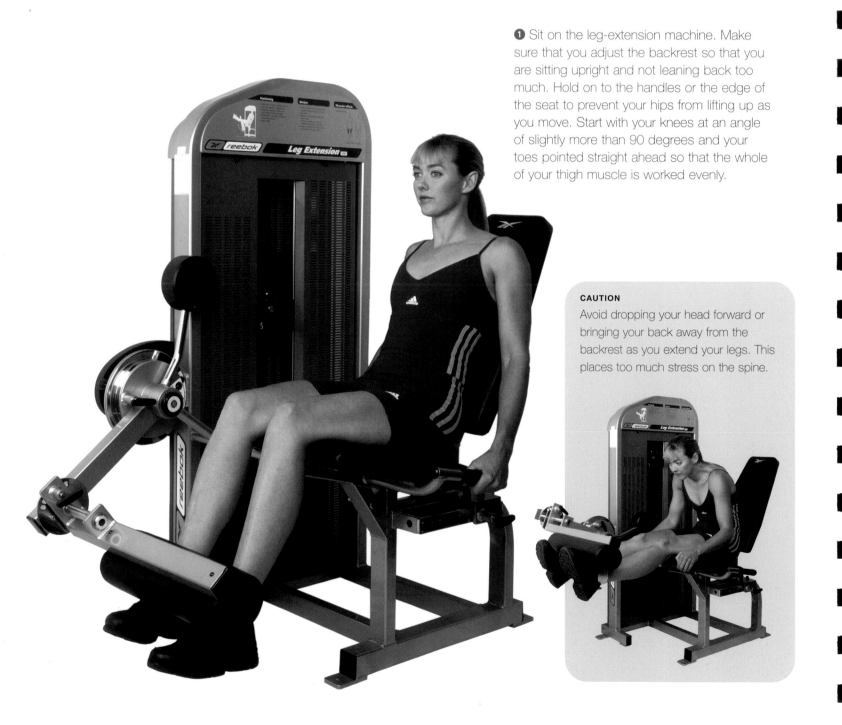

❶ Sit on the leg-extension machine. Make sure that you adjust the backrest so that you are sitting upright and not leaning back too much. Hold on to the handles or the edge of the seat to prevent your hips from lifting up as you move. Start with your knees at an angle of slightly more than 90 degrees and your toes pointed straight ahead so that the whole of your thigh muscle is worked evenly.

CAUTION

Avoid dropping your head forward or bringing your back away from the backrest as you extend your legs. This places too much stress on the spine.

❷ Slowly lift your ankles, straightening your legs but keeping your knees slightly bent. Hold for a count of one, then slowly lower the weight to the starting position, with your knees at an angle of a little more than 90 degrees. Lowering the weight any farther could place too much stress on the knee joint, leading to injury and knee pain.

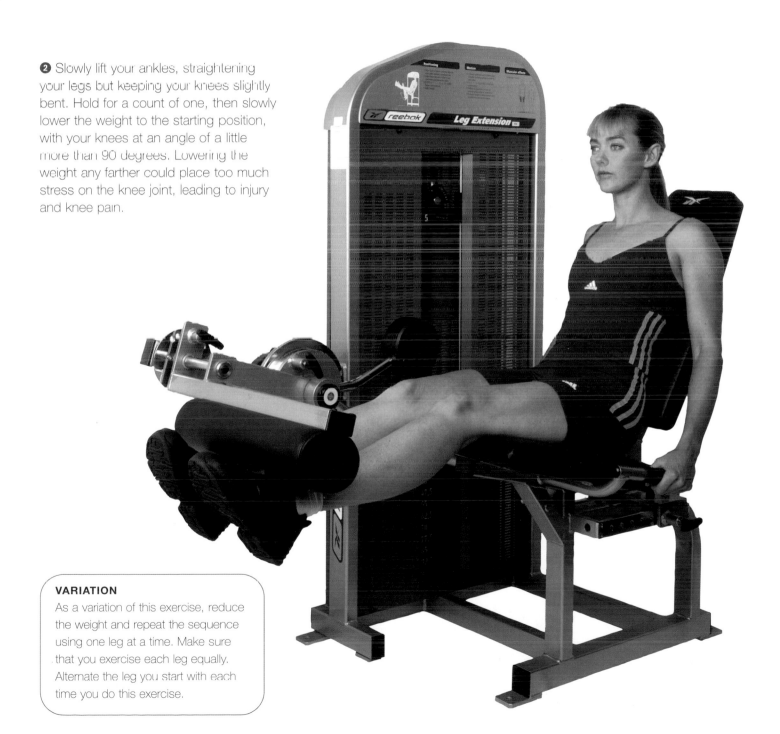

VARIATION

As a variation of this exercise, reduce the weight and repeat the sequence using one leg at a time. Make sure that you exercise each leg equally. Alternate the leg you start with each time you do this exercise.

dumbbell step-ups

This is an exercise that can be done anywhere there is a high platform such as a box, a bench top, a small wall, a high ledge, or even a few steps. It can be done with or without dumbbells in your hands.

level: beginner

main muscles worked: quadriceps

secondary muscles worked: glutes, hamstrings, calves

equipment used: bench or platform, dumbbells

type of exercise: isolation

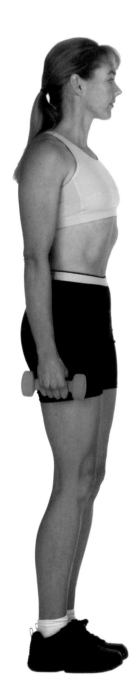

❶ Stand up tall with your back straight and your eyes focused straight ahead. Your legs should be positioned approximately hip width apart, feet parallel and pointing straight ahead. If you wish to use weights here, hold one dumbbell in each hand, palms facing inward, arms by your sides.

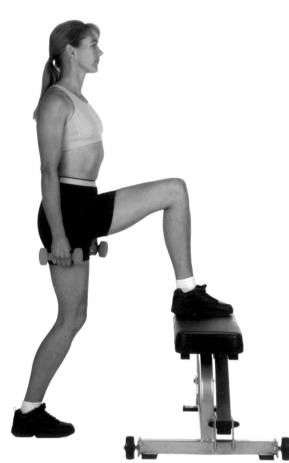

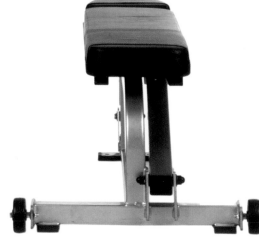

❷ Slowly step up onto the bench or other stable platform with your right foot, making sure that your whole foot is placed firmly on the bench. Then immediately step up with your left foot, so that you are standing on the bench. Take your time. If you rush through this exercise you might lose your balance and fall.

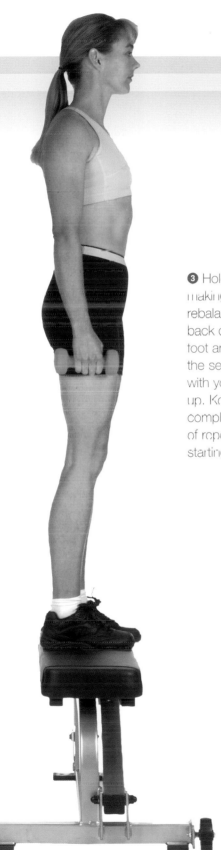

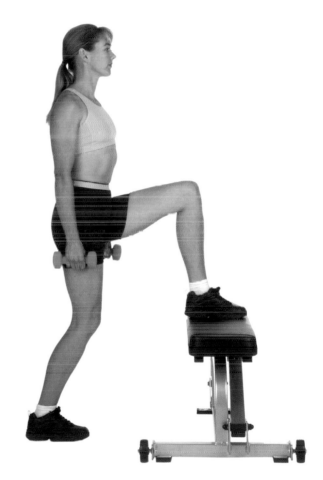

3 Hold for a count of one, making sure that you have rebalanced yourself, then step back down, first with your left foot and then your right. Repeat the sequence, this time leading with your left foot as you step up. Keep going until you have completed the desired number of repetitions, changing the starting foot each time.

CAUTION

• Maintain a slow and controlled rhythm as you step.

• Avoid rushing, or you may lose your concentration and your balance.

• Make sure you plant your feet firmly on the bench and floor with each step. If you do find that you are wobbling from side to side, practice the exercise without dumbbells until your stability and muscle control improves. Learning how to perform the step-up exercise correctly and with control is much more important than struggling to do it with a dumbbell in each hand.

Swiss-ball squats

Beginners can benefit from this exercise because it is one of the easiest free-standing squat exercises to learn. It is also good for intermediate strength trainers because it demands a certain level of strength in your lumbar spine and leg muscles to stabilize yourself as you move. The ball acts as a back support and keeps your upper body straight.

level: beginner–intermediate

main muscles worked: quadriceps

secondary muscles worked: glutes, lower back, hamstrings, calves, abdominals

equipment used: Swiss ball

type of exercise: size (mass)-building

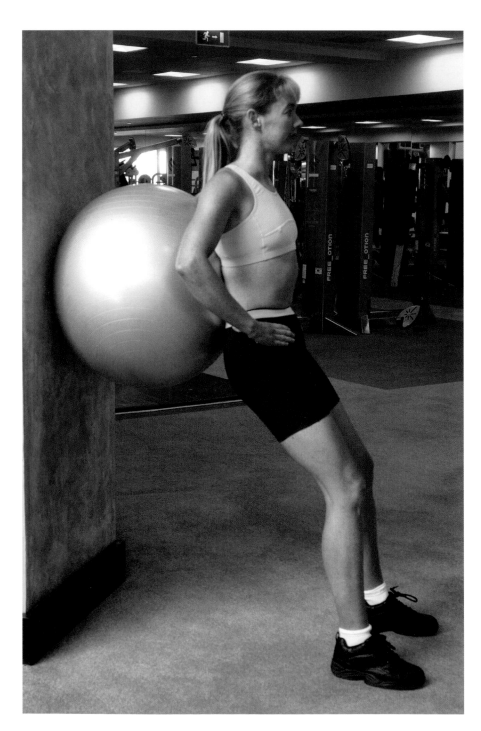

❶ Place the Swiss ball between the middle of your back and the wall. If you have difficulty getting into position you might want to have someone else to help you. Your body should be upright with your eyes focused straight ahead and your feet approximately hip width apart with toes pointing forward. Hands should be on your hips or lightly resting on the tops of your thighs for support.

CAUTION
Avoid placing your feet too far back toward the wall or too far forward, as this might cause you to lose your balance and fall. Also be careful of rolling too far down the wall with the Swiss ball—you could lose your balance or injure your neck.

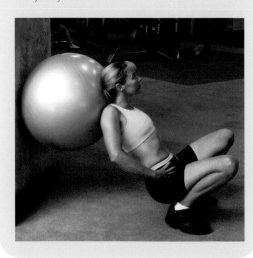

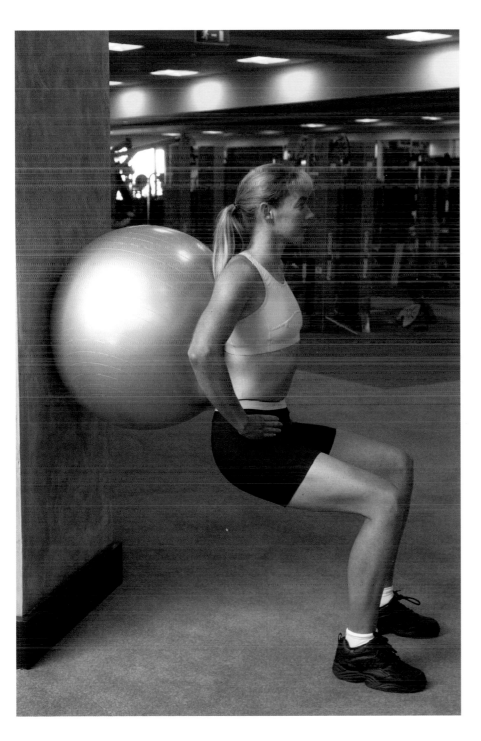

❷ Once in position, your legs should be almost straight (with a slight bend in the knees). Inhale and slowly lower your body until your thighs are parallel to the floor. If you are unable to lower yourself this far, just go as far as is comfortable until your strength and stability improves and you are able to work yourself all the way down to the parallel position.

❸ Hold for a count of one, then exhale and slowly raise yourself to the starting position, keeping your torso upright.

standing bench crossovers

Essentially this is the same movement as the dumbbell step-ups (page 132), except that here you are standing next to the bench rather than facing it. This movement can be done in the gym, at home, or outside and can be performed with or without dumbbells.

level: beginner

main muscles worked: quadriceps

secondary muscles worked: glutes, hamstrings, calves

equipment used: bench

type of exercise: isolation

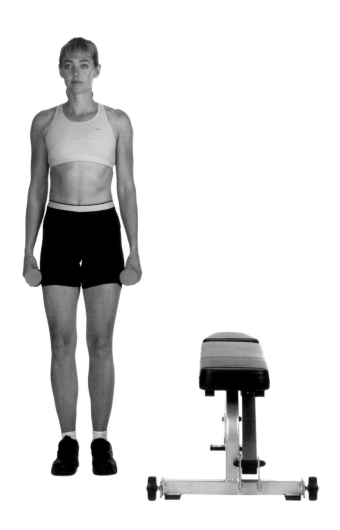
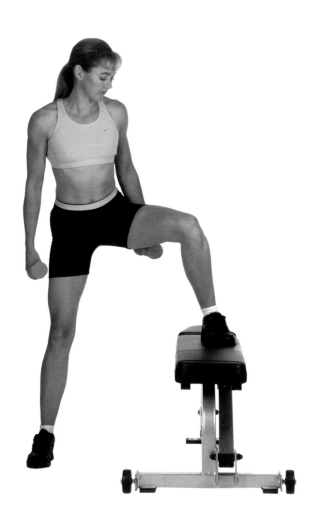

❶ Stand to the right of the bench with your feet close together, parallel to the bench. Stand with your back straight and your eyes looking straight ahead, preferably into a mirror so that you can monitor what you are doing. If there is no mirror to guide you, be careful; it is easy to step over the bench or miss it completely. Your arms should hang loosely by your sides throughout.

❷ Step up onto the bench first with your left foot and then your right, so you are standing on the bench.

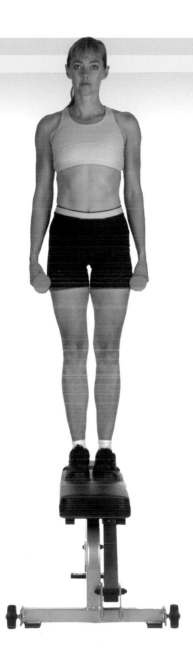

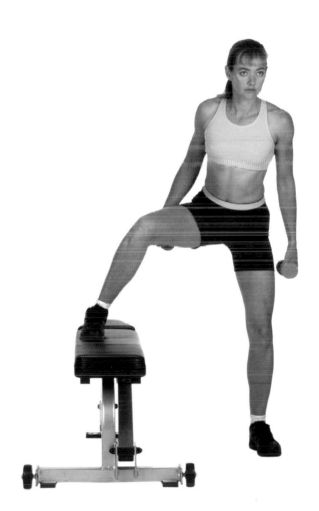

❸ Stand fully upright on the bench for a count of one while you rebalance yourself, then step down off the bench on the opposite side, first with your left foot and then your right. Repeat by stepping on the bench with your right foot this time, and continue the exercise for the desired amount of repetitions.

CAUTION

• Maintain a slow and controlled rhythm as you step. Avoid rushing as you step up or down, which could cause you to lose your concentration and your balance.

• Plant your feet firmly on the floor and bench each time you step. If you find that you are wobbling from side to side, try holding your arms straight out to your sides, parallel with your shoulders, to help you balance.

stationary dumbbell forward lunges

This is a challenging exercise to do even without any added resistance from dumbbells.

level: intermediate

main muscles worked: quadriceps

secondary muscles worked: hamstrings, calves, glutes

equipment used: dumbbells

type of exercise: isolation

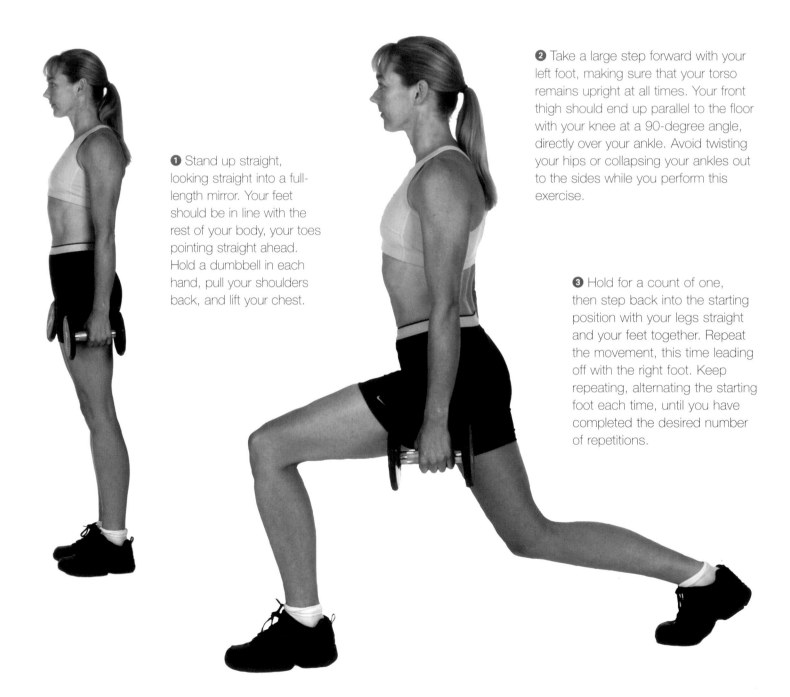

❶ Stand up straight, looking straight into a full-length mirror. Your feet should be in line with the rest of your body, your toes pointing straight ahead. Hold a dumbbell in each hand, pull your shoulders back, and lift your chest.

❷ Take a large step forward with your left foot, making sure that your torso remains upright at all times. Your front thigh should end up parallel to the floor with your knee at a 90-degree angle, directly over your ankle. Avoid twisting your hips or collapsing your ankles out to the sides while you perform this exercise.

❸ Hold for a count of one, then step back into the starting position with your legs straight and your feet together. Repeat the movement, this time leading off with the right foot. Keep repeating, alternating the starting foot each time, until you have completed the desired number of repetitions.

CAUTION

• Avoid taking your knee too far forward—it should not be past your toes—as this places too much stress on the knee joint.

• Try not to look at the floor as you perform this exercise; this will encourage you to lean over and lose the correct posture.

• If you find that you are unable to balance yourself as you move, practice without weights and hold your arms straight out to the sides and parallel to the ground to help you balance.

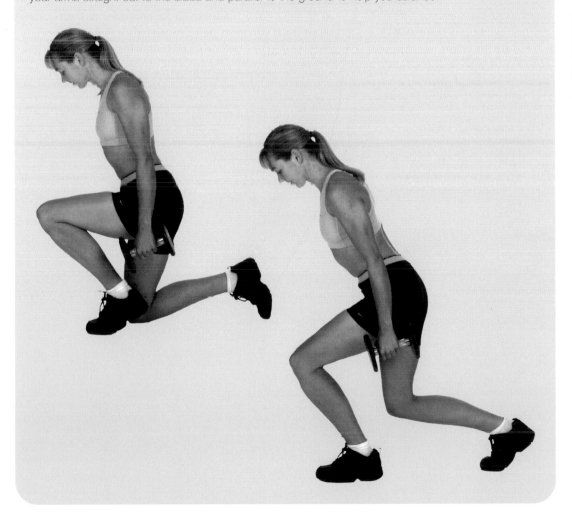

VARIATIONS

There are many variations of the lunge exercise—it can be done standing in one position, taking your legs either forward or backward; it can be performed with dumbbells or using a bar, machine, or medicine ball. My favorite type of lunge is the walking lunge. This can be done either indoors or outdoors across a park or along a straight path.

• Before you attempt any variations, it is essential that you learn to do the basic movement correctly.

seated machine thigh abductor

Many women feel that they suffer from lack of shape around the outer thighs. The outer thighs are tough to work effectively, but the added resistance of the weight in the abductor machine places the muscle under enough stress to tone, shape, and define your thighs.

level: beginner

main muscles worked: quadriceps

secondary muscles worked: hamstrings, abductor muscle (also known as the abductor longus) on the outside of your thighs

equipment used: hip-abduction machine

type of exercise: isolation

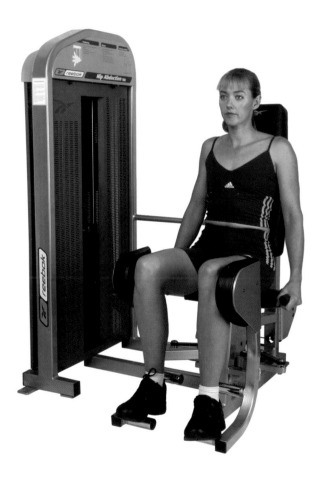 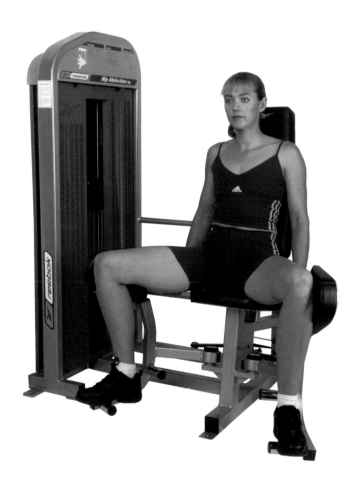

❶ Sit upright with your back firmly against the backrest. Keep your eyes focused straight ahead throughout the movement. Place your feet on the footrests with the pads positioned against your thighs and close to your knees.

CAUTION

• Open your legs only as far as is comfortable; otherwise you risk causing strain to the hips and may find that you start to arch your back. Remember to keep your upper body firmly on the backrest with your head facing forward—looking down while performing this exercise places stress on your neck.

• Make sure that you control the weight as you bring your legs back in to the center.

❷ Slowly push against the thigh pads and open your legs to a comfortable distance.

❸ Hold for a count of one before slowly bringing your legs back to center. Repeat.

sealed machine thigh adductor

This movement is the reverse of the abductor machine—here you're squeezing your thighs together rather than pushing them apart. Now you're working that all-important, hard-to-tone inner-thigh area.

level: beginner

main muscles worked: quadriceps

secondary muscles worked: hamstrings, adductor muscle (also known as the adductor magnus) on the inside of your thighs

equipment used: hip-adduction machine

type of exercise: isolation

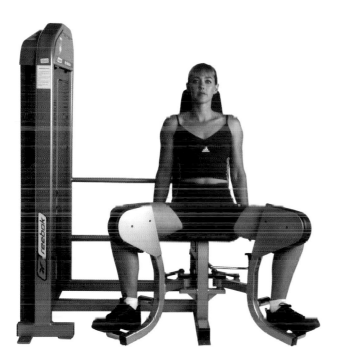

strength tip
Over 50 percent of sports injuries (in many types of sports) are due to weak inner-thigh muscles. The inner thigh is one of the most neglected areas in strength training and one of the most vital areas to work.

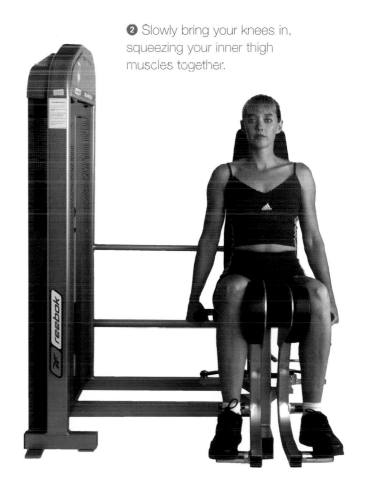

❷ Slowly bring your knees in, squeezing your inner thigh muscles together.

❶ Sit with your back firmly against the backrest. Keep your eyes focused straight ahead throughout this movement. Place your feet on the footrests with the pads positioned against your thighs and close to your knees. Open your legs to a comfortable position before starting the movement.

CAUTION

• As with the abductor exercise, remember to keep your back firmly in contact with the backrest and your head facing straight forward; avoid looking down and placing pressure on your neck.

• As you release your legs outward, make sure you control the move with your thigh muscles—avoid simply letting go and allowing the machine to take over.

❸ Hold for a count of one and then slowly release, controlling the move as you open your legs back to the starting position. Repeat.

hamstrings

Also known as: biceps femoris, hamstring tendon, hams, thigh biceps, posterior thigh muscles

When thinking of shapely, toned legs, we tend to think of the thighs, but for overall strength and shape we need to also remember the muscles behind the quadriceps, the hamstrings. Toned hamstrings give a natural sweep to the legs and help to create a separation line that runs from the hip to the knee joint. This separation line creates a division between the thigh muscles and the hamstring.

Technically, the hamstring consists of three main sections: the semimembranosus, the semitendinosus, and the biceps femoris muscles (long head and short head). In strength training we try to isolate these three sections in order to create well-rounded thigh biceps.

The main functions of the hamstrings are to bend (flex) the knee, and to straighten (extend) the hip as the thigh moves backward. Interestingly enough, the hamstrings are not actively involved with many normal daily movements such as sitting or walking. Nevertheless, they are very involved when it comes to movements or exercises that demand any kind of power, such as running, rock climbing, sprinting, and jumping. So, for the average person it is entirely possible to get through daily activities with very weak hamstrings. But for those who are very active, strong, well-conditioned hamstrings are essential.

Hamstring injuries are very common, particularly for those people who suffer from tight hamstrings, neglect to warm up sufficiently, or do not regularly include any stretching in their exercise routine. If the opposing muscle group (quadriceps) is stronger than the hamstring for any reason, the imbalance of strength between the two muscles can cause unnecessary strain on the weaker muscle. Just like in a tug of war game, if the contestants on one side are stronger, they'll end up undermining the strength of the opposing team and cause them to fall flat on their faces. The same is true for flexibility. At some time or other, most of us have complained of pain and a feeling of tightness in the back of the thigh. Just like an elastic band, if your hamstrings are too tight, it can lead to an ache, a strain, or even a tear in the muscle. To minimize the risk or even prevent such injuries from occurring, regular stretching and strength-training exercises that specifically target the hamstrings are essential.

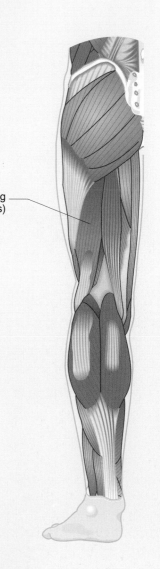

Hamstring
(biceps femoris)

seated leg curls

This exercise is easier to master than the lying leg curls (page 146) and is more comfortable, too, although it is equally effective in working the hamstrings. The movement itself is the reverse of the seated leg extensions for the thigh muscles. It can be done as either a double-leg or a single-leg exercise.

level: beginner

main muscles worked: hamstrings

secondary muscles worked: none

equipment used: leg-curl machine

type of exercise: isolation

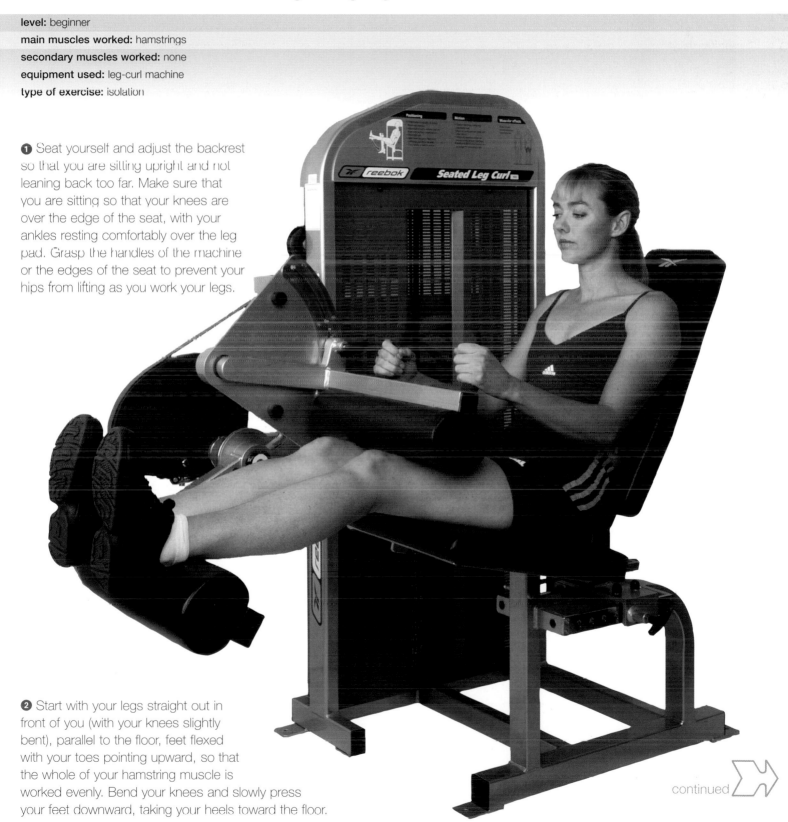

❶ Seat yourself and adjust the backrest so that you are sitting upright and not leaning back too far. Make sure that you are sitting so that your knees are over the edge of the seat, with your ankles resting comfortably over the leg pad. Grasp the handles of the machine or the edges of the seat to prevent your hips from lifting as you work your legs.

❷ Start with your legs straight out in front of you (with your knees slightly bent), parallel to the floor, feet flexed with your toes pointing upward, so that the whole of your hamstring muscle is worked evenly. Bend your knees and slowly press your feet downward, taking your heels toward the floor.

continued ⟩⟩

seated leg curls (continued)

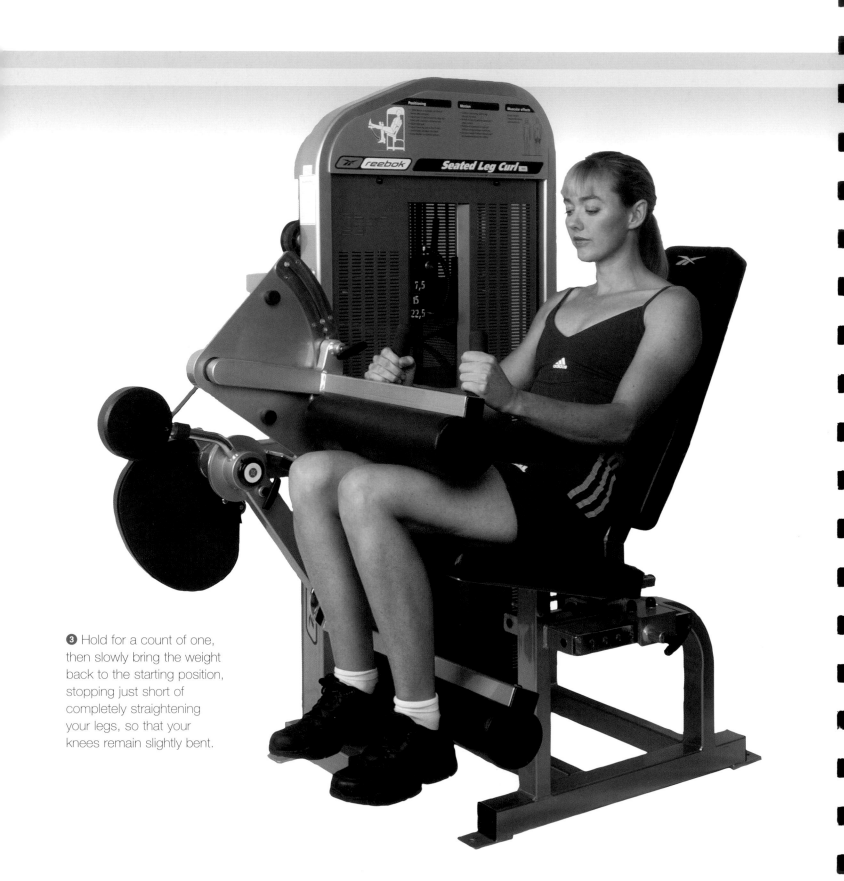

❸ Hold for a count of one, then slowly bring the weight back to the starting position, stopping just short of completely straightening your legs, so that your knees remain slightly bent.

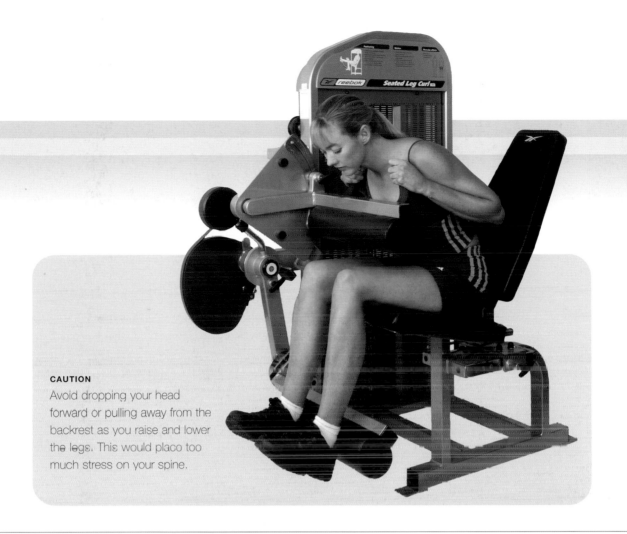

CAUTION

Avoid dropping your head forward or pulling away from the backrest as you raise and lower the legs. This would place too much stress on your spine.

VARIATION

As a variation of this exercise, reduce the weight and repeat the sequence using one leg at a time, making sure that you exercise each leg equally. Try to alternate the leg you start with each time you perform this single-leg version of the exercise.

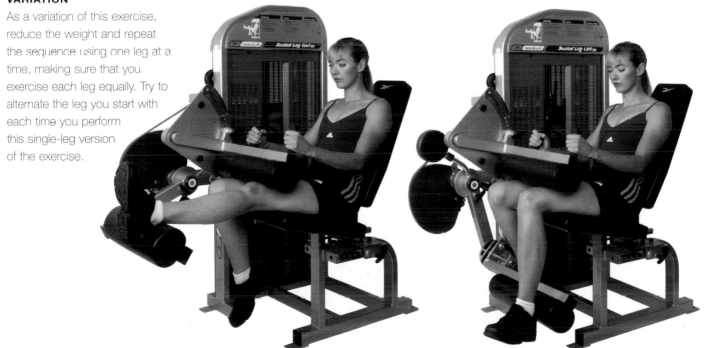

lying leg curls

This exercise effectively isolates the hamstring muscle, giving shape and tone to the back of the thigh. However, not everyone finds this facedown exercise comfortable—if you are overweight or have a particularly large bust, I would suggest omitting this exercise from your routine and concentrating on the seated leg curl instead.

level: beginner

main muscles worked: hamstrings

secondary muscles worked: none

equipment used: leg-curl machine

type of exercise: isolation

❶ Adjust the leg roller pad so that it rests on your ankles, then lie facedown on the leg-curl machine and hook your ankles under the roller pad. While keeping your hips and upper body flat on the bench, grasp the machine handles on either side of you for support.

❷ Without lifting your head up (you should keep facing down toward the bench) or moving your body off the bench, slowly raise your heels toward your buttocks as far as you can. Ideally, you should aim to curl the weight to the point where the pad momentarily touches your butt.

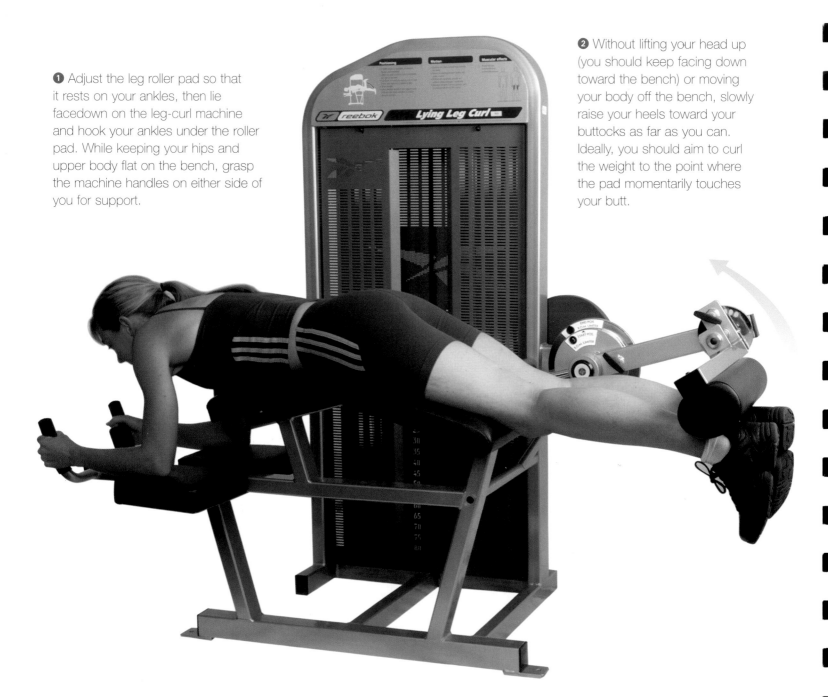

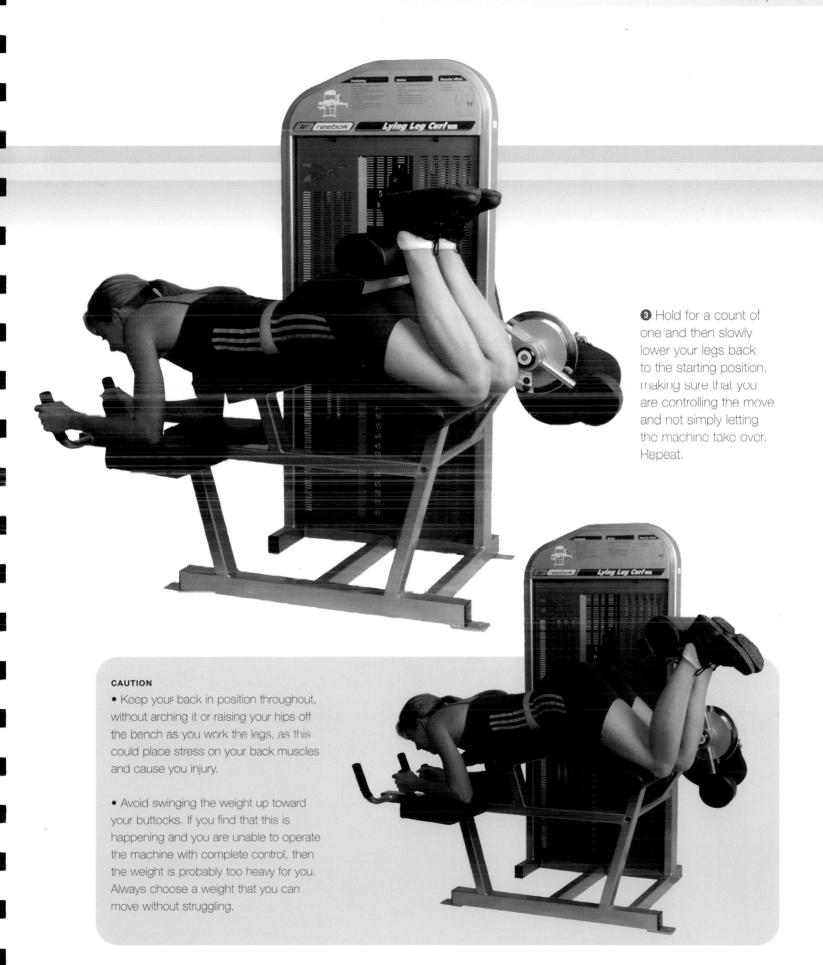

❸ Hold for a count of one and then slowly lower your legs back to the starting position, making sure that you are controlling the move and not simply letting the machine take over. Repeat.

CAUTION

• Keep your back in position throughout, without arching it or raising your hips off the bench as you work the legs, as this could place stress on your back muscles and cause you injury.

• Avoid swinging the weight up toward your buttocks. If you find that this is happening and you are unable to operate the machine with complete control, then the weight is probably too heavy for you. Always choose a weight that you can move without struggling.

glutes

Also known as: gluteus maximus, gluteus muscles, gluteal muscles, buttocks, butt

Improving the shape and tone of the buttocks seems to be a priority in most strength-training routines for women.

The buttocks are made up of three major muscles. These are the gluteus maximus, the gluteus medius, and the gluteus minimus. Glute exercises isolate these three muscles, allowing you to work at gradually creating a well-toned bottom.

The glute muscles play a fundamental role in all aspects of posture and motion, such as standing erect, walking, running, climbing stairs, rising from a chair, or going up hills. They also work hard in movements such as bending forward, squatting, and lunging with the legs. Whatever movement you do with your lower legs, you will always somehow, directly or indirectly, be working your buttock muscles.

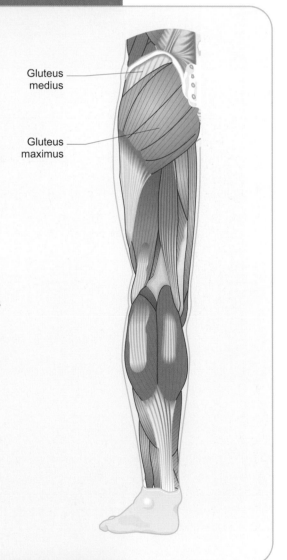

Gluteus medius

Gluteus maximus

glute machine raises

This is an extremely intense exercise when performed using a glute machine, although it can be just as effective when performed as a simple floor exercise.

level: beginner
main muscles worked: glutes
secondary muscles worked: hamstrings
equipment used: glute raises machine
type of exercise: isolation

❶ Position the knee pad and chest pad so that you can lie comfortably with your upper body parallel to the floor and your knees at 90 degrees. Support yourself with your elbows on the elbow pads while holding the handles to either side.

CAUTION
Make sure that your upper body remains parallel to the floor throughout, with your head in line with the rest of your body and your neck relaxed. If you lift your head as you work the legs, you'll place unnecessary stress on your neck muscles.

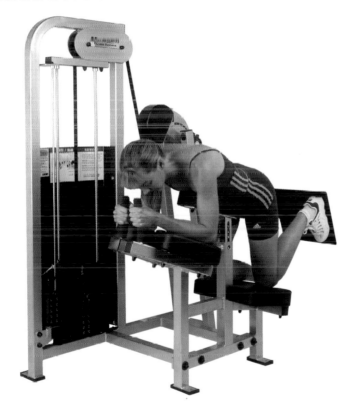

❸ Hold for a count of one, then slowly lower your foot to the starting position, still squeezing your buttocks. When you have completed the desired number of repetitions, switch legs and repeat the sequence for the other side.

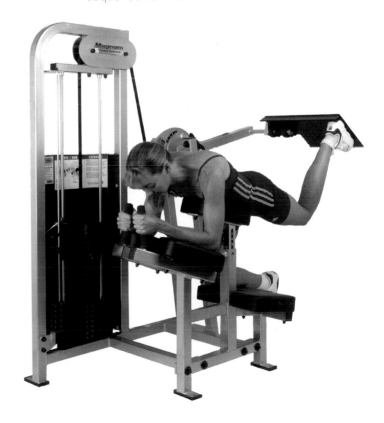

❷ With your left foot resting on the machine platform (or the machine pad behind the back of your knee, depending on what type of glute machine you are using), squeeze your buttocks and slowly raise your left foot up toward the ceiling until your thigh is parallel to the floor.

glute body raises

This is an excellent exercise for toning the pelvic muscles as well as the glutes. This exercise should be performed on a fairly soft surface, such as an exercise mat or a folded blanket, to give your back support.

level: beginner
main muscles worked: glutes
secondary muscles worked: hamstrings, pelvic muscles
equipment used: mat
type of exercise: isolation

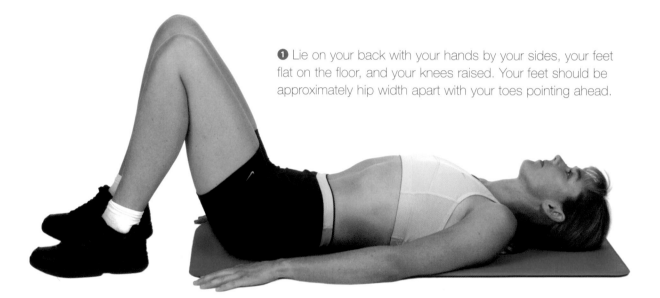

❶ Lie on your back with your hands by your sides, your feet flat on the floor, and your knees raised. Your feet should be approximately hip width apart with your toes pointing ahead.

❷ Squeeze your buttocks and lift your hips up off the floor until your body is in a straight line, like a mini ski slope. Keep your back straight at all times so that the movement is entirely from the hips and pelvic area.

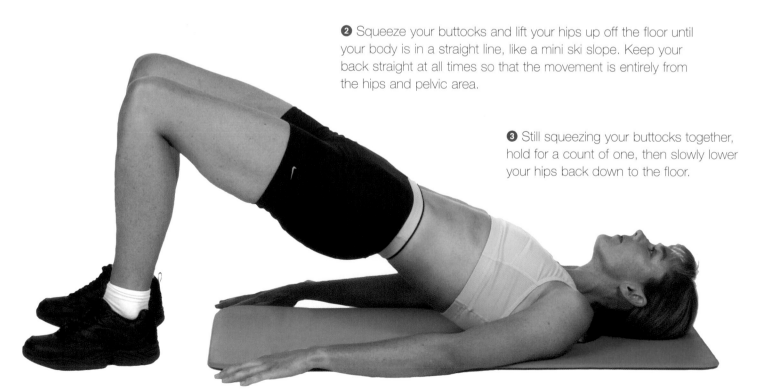

❸ Still squeezing your buttocks together, hold for a count of one, then slowly lower your hips back down to the floor.

CAUTION

Avoid letting your upper body sink into the floor as you lower your hips; this can place unnecessary stress on your neck muscles.

VARIATION

For a slightly more challenging version of this exercise, try resting your ankles on a bench or box as you work.

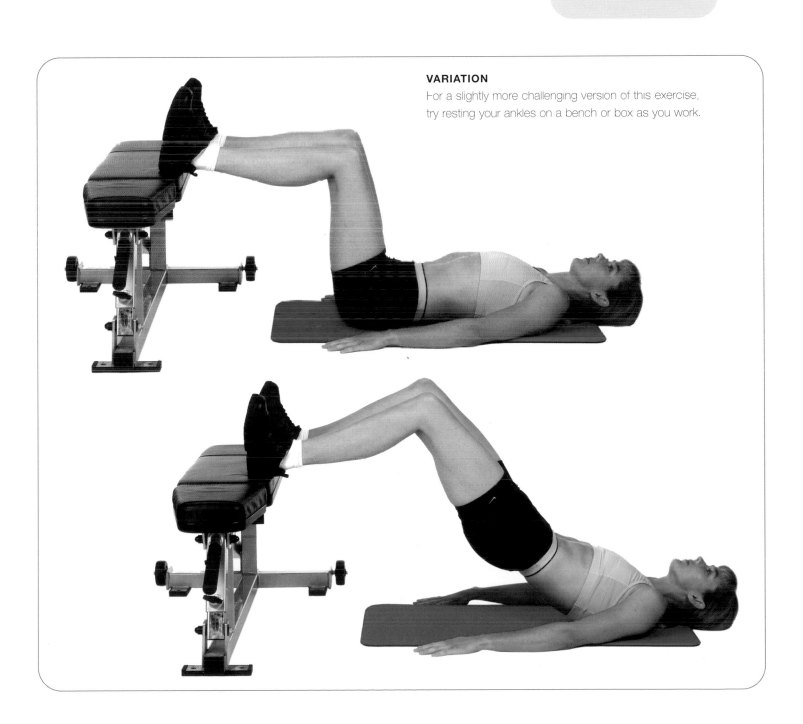

glute kickbacks

This is exactly the same movement as the glute machine raises but without the additional weight and resistance provided by the machine. This version is still extremely effective, particularly if performed in a slow and controlled manner.

level: beginner
main muscles worked: glutes
secondary muscles worked: hamstrings
equipment used: mat
type of exercise: isolation

❶ Kneel on a mat on the floor on all fours, with your hands approximately shoulder width apart and your knees directly below your hips. (For a slightly easier version, give yourself a little more stability by placing your forearms on the floor with your elbows directly below your shoulders and your hands pointing forward, as pictured.)

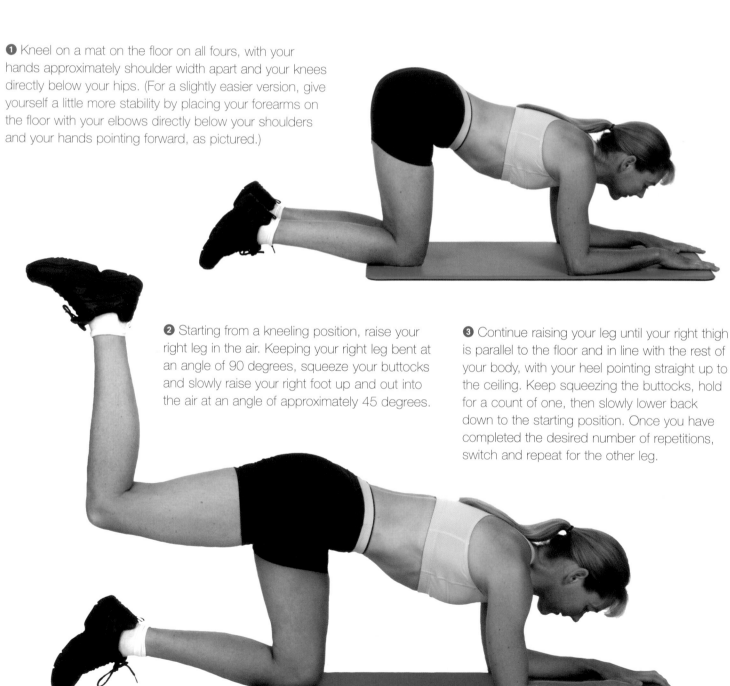

❷ Starting from a kneeling position, raise your right leg in the air. Keeping your right leg bent at an angle of 90 degrees, squeeze your buttocks and slowly raise your right foot up and out into the air at an angle of approximately 45 degrees.

❸ Continue raising your leg until your right thigh is parallel to the floor and in line with the rest of your body, with your heel pointing straight up to the ceiling. Keep squeezing the buttocks, hold for a count of one, then slowly lower back down to the starting position. Once you have completed the desired number of repetitions, switch and repeat for the other leg.

strength tip
In some ways, this exercise can be more demanding when done as a floor exercise; you need to have more stability and better muscle control when you don't have the machine to help you. You will almost certainly have come across this exercise if you've taken any gym classes that focused on the glutes and thighs.

CAUTION
• Keep your back straight and your body parallel to the floor, with your head and neck in line with the rest of your body. If you lift your head as you raise and lower your legs, you'll place too much strain on your neck muscles.

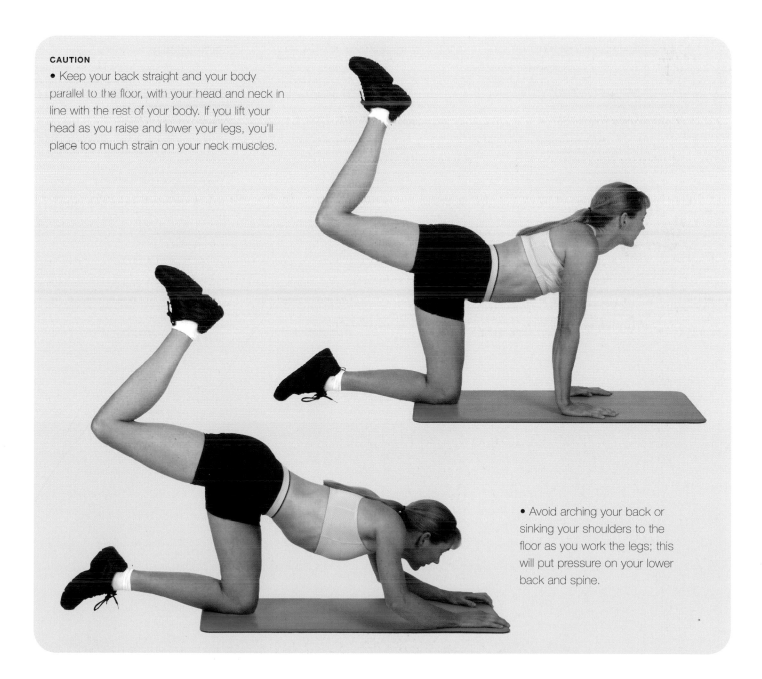

• Avoid arching your back or sinking your shoulders to the floor as you work the legs; this will put pressure on your lower back and spine.

calves

Also known as: gastrocnemius muscle

What's the point of having fantastic upper-leg shape and tone if you don't work the all-important area below the knees—your calves? Whether you wear heels or flat shoes, well-rounded calves add that extra pizzazz to the back of your leg.

The calf muscles include the gastrocnemius and the soleus. The gastrocnemius is the main calf muscle and gives the calf its strong, rounded shape. The soleus is a flat muscle running underneath the gastrocnemius.

The main function of the calf muscle is to point the toe forward, to allow you to stand on your toes, to run, jump, walk, and climb up and down stairs. Strong, well-shaped calves are essential in everyday life, as they are less prone to injury and unnecessary muscle tightness that could lead to strain, pain, and, in more serious cases, muscle tear.

Tight calves seem to be a common problem among women who regularly wear very high heels, and for those who are not in the habit of exercising, or omit regular stretching from their exercise routine. Weak calf muscles can easily be improved through strength-training exercises that specifically target the calf area.

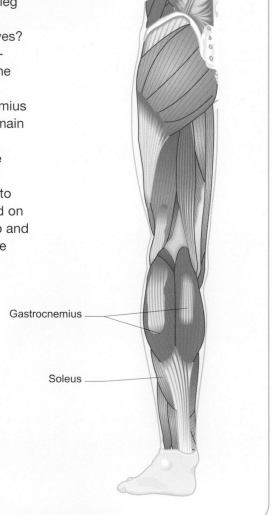

Gastrocnemius

Soleus

standing machine calf raises

I believe this is the number-one exercise for overall calf development, shape, and tone. If you have access to a gym I would certainly recommend using the standing calf machine. If you are exercising at home or would like to add some variety to your exercises, this movement can be done holding a dumbbell in each hand and standing on a stair or step.

level: beginner

main muscles worked: gastrocnemius and soleus muscles

secondary muscles worked: none

equipment used: standing calf machine

type of exercise: isolation

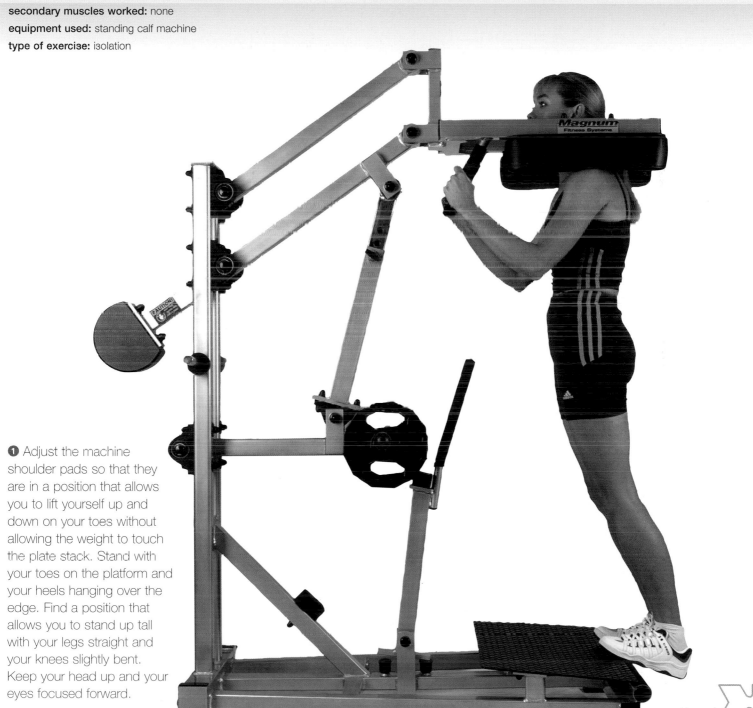

❶ Adjust the machine shoulder pads so that they are in a position that allows you to lift yourself up and down on your toes without allowing the weight to touch the plate stack. Stand with your toes on the platform and your heels hanging over the edge. Find a position that allows you to stand up tall with your legs straight and your knees slightly bent. Keep your head up and your eyes focused forward.

continued

standing machine calf raises (continued)

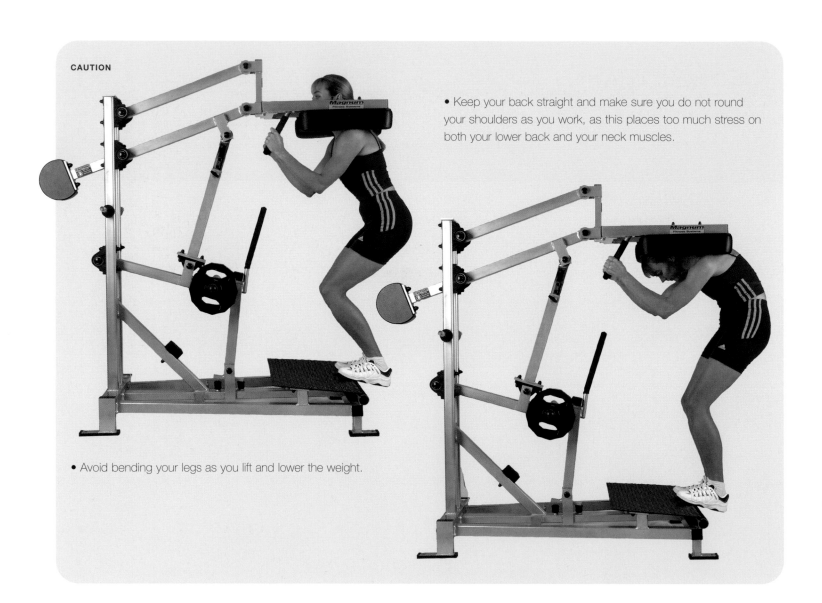

CAUTION

• Keep your back straight and make sure you do not round your shoulders as you work, as this places too much stress on both your lower back and your neck muscles.

• Avoid bending your legs as you lift and lower the weight.

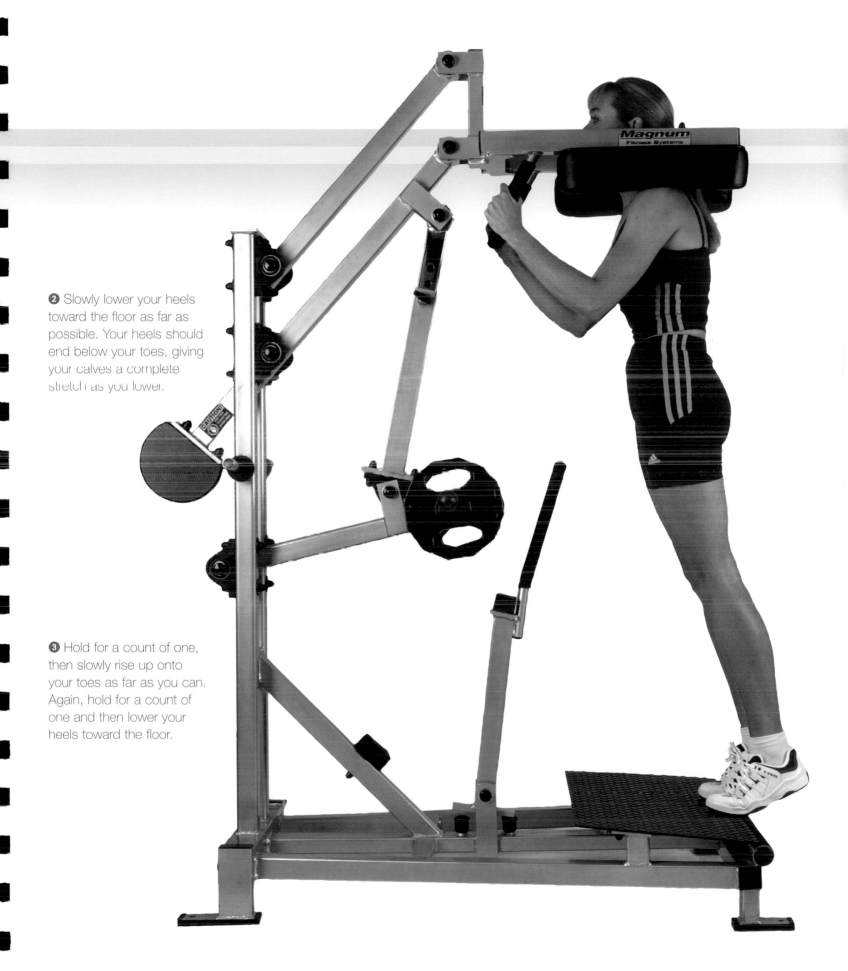

❷ Slowly lower your heels toward the floor as far as possible. Your heels should end below your toes, giving your calves a complete stretch as you lower.

❸ Hold for a count of one, then slowly rise up onto your toes as far as you can. Again, hold for a count of one and then lower your heels toward the floor.

one-leg standing calf raises

This exercise can be done on a step or stair, a step platform (used for step classes), or a raised platform (two to three inches high)—any raised area that will not slip as you move and is deep enough to allow you to fully stretch your calf muscle at the bottom and top of the movement.

level: beginner

main muscles worked: gastrocnemius and soleus muscles

secondary muscles worked: none

equipment used: step, dumbbell

type of exercise: isolation

❶ Position yourself on a step or stair with the toes of your left foot on the step and your heel hanging over the edge. Hold a dumbbell in your left hand and lift your right leg away from the ground, using your right arm to help you balance by holding on to a wall or rail for support. Keep your body straight and your head up, eyes looking straight ahead.

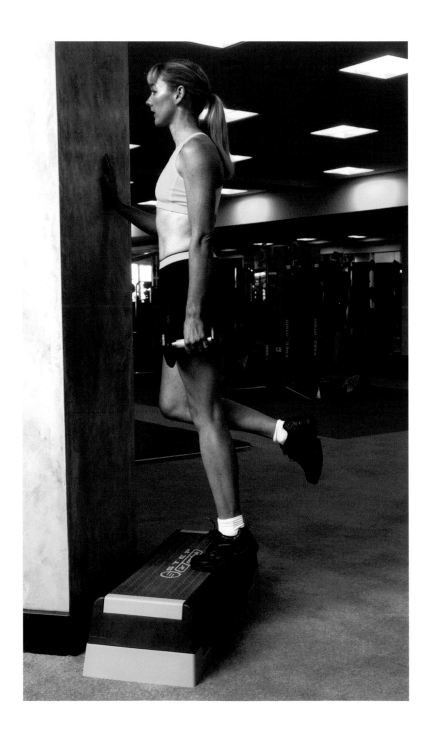

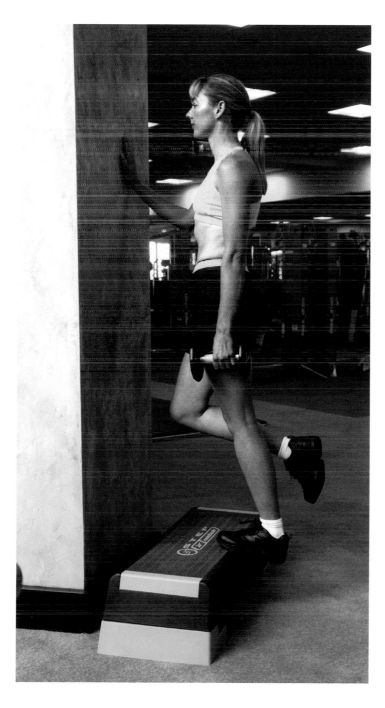

❷ Keeping your left leg straight with the knee slightly bent, lower your left heel as far as possible toward the floor. Hold the rail or wall firmly with your right hand so that you don't lose your balance or fall backward as you work.

❸ Hold for a count of one, then slowly rise up on your left toes as high as you can. Again, hold for a count of one, then lower your heel toward the floor again. Complete the desired number of repetitions, then switch legs and repeat for the other side.

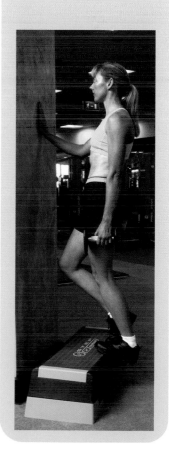

seated calf raises

This exercise is different from the standing machine calf raise (which works both the gastrocnemius and the soleus muscles) in that it specifically targets the soleus—the smaller muscle that is located lower down in the leg, running underneath the gastrocnemius.

level: beginner

main muscles worked: soleus muscles

secondary muscles worked: none

equipment used: bench, weight plate, step platform

type of exercise: isolation

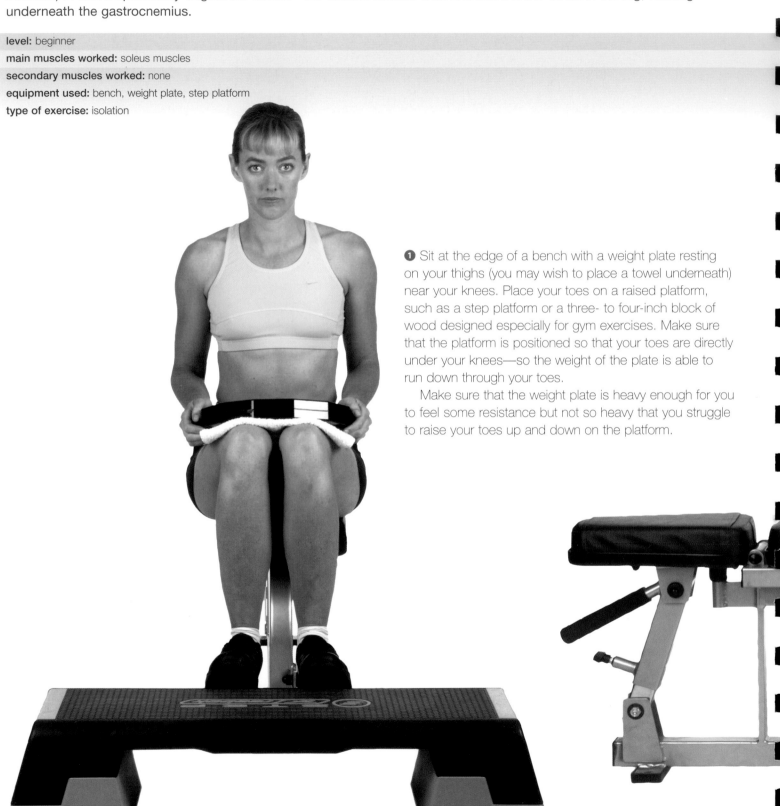

❶ Sit at the edge of a bench with a weight plate resting on your thighs (you may wish to place a towel underneath) near your knees. Place your toes on a raised platform, such as a step platform or a three- to four-inch block of wood designed especially for gym exercises. Make sure that the platform is positioned so that your toes are directly under your knees—so the weight of the plate is able to run down through your toes.

Make sure that the weight plate is heavy enough for you to feel some resistance but not so heavy that you struggle to raise your toes up and down on the platform.

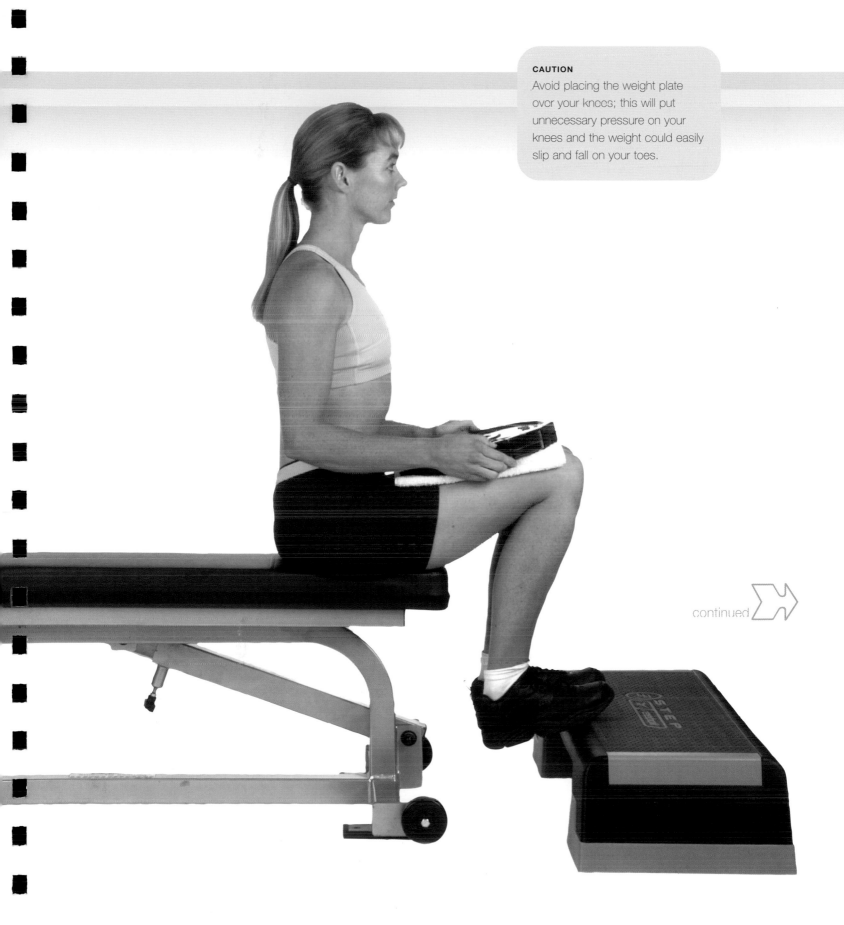

continued

CAUTION

Avoid placing the weight plate over your knees; this will put unnecessary pressure on your knees and the weight could easily slip and fall on your toes.

seated calf raises (continued)

strength tip
To achieve overall development, shape, and tone in the calf muscles, it is essential to target all the different parts of the muscles from every angle using a range of exercises, including the seated calf raise.

❷ Holding the weight plate on your lap to keep it from slipping forward and falling, slowly rise upward onto your toes as high as you can (as pictured at left and at right).

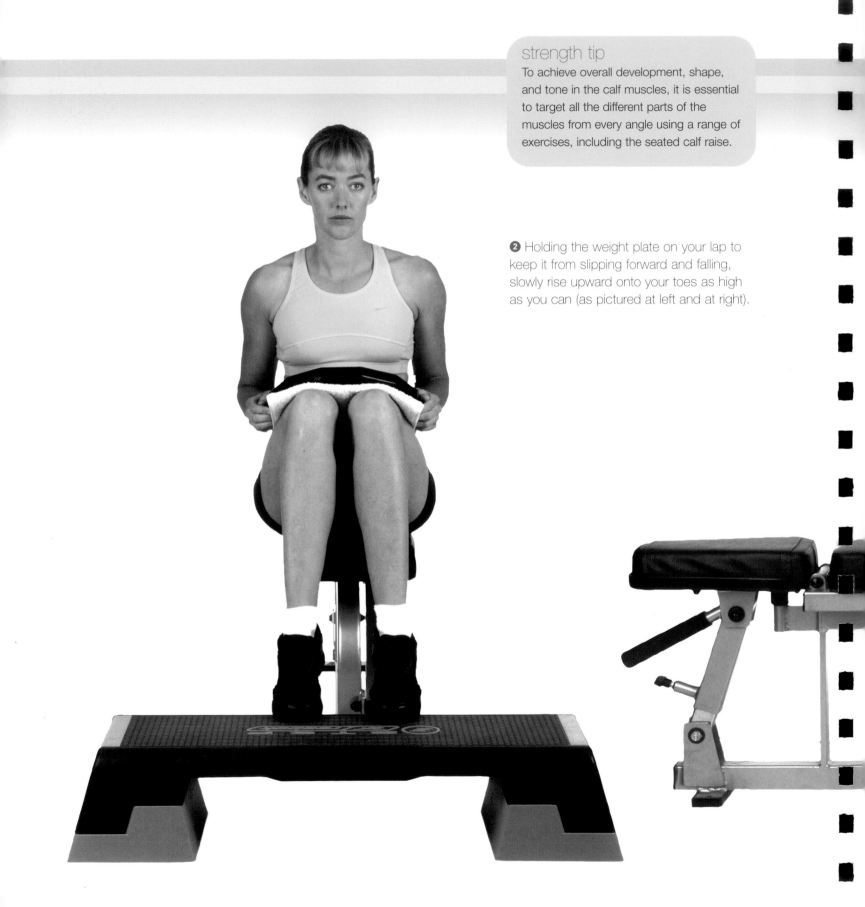

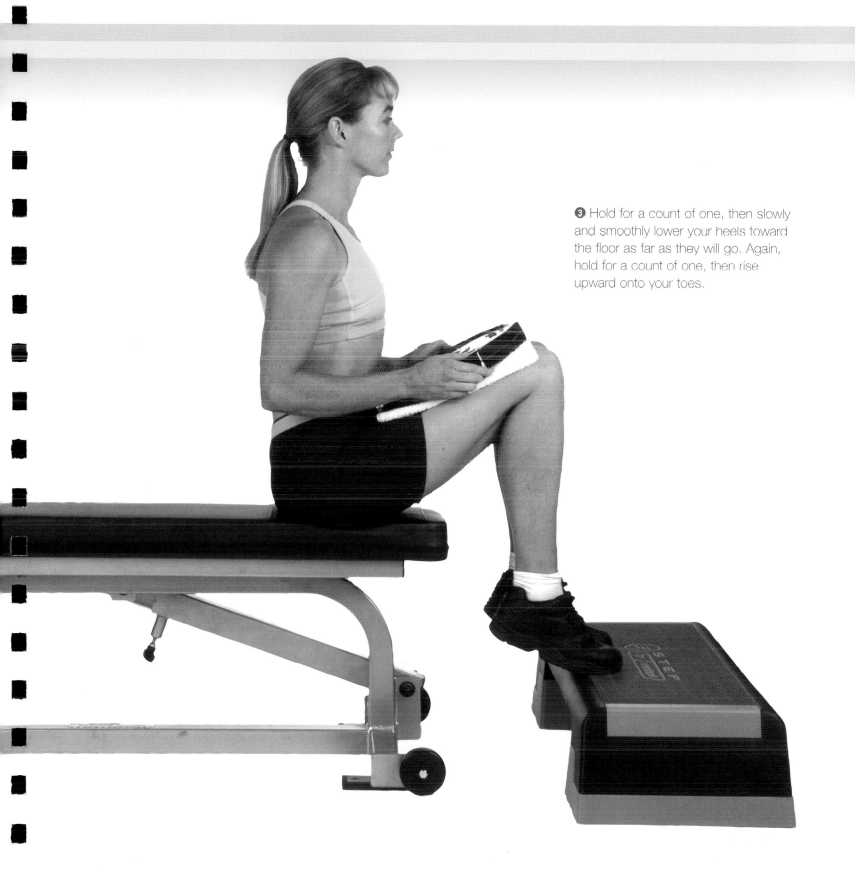

3 Hold for a count of one, then slowly and smoothly lower your heels toward the floor as far as they will go. Again, hold for a count of one, then rise upward onto your toes.

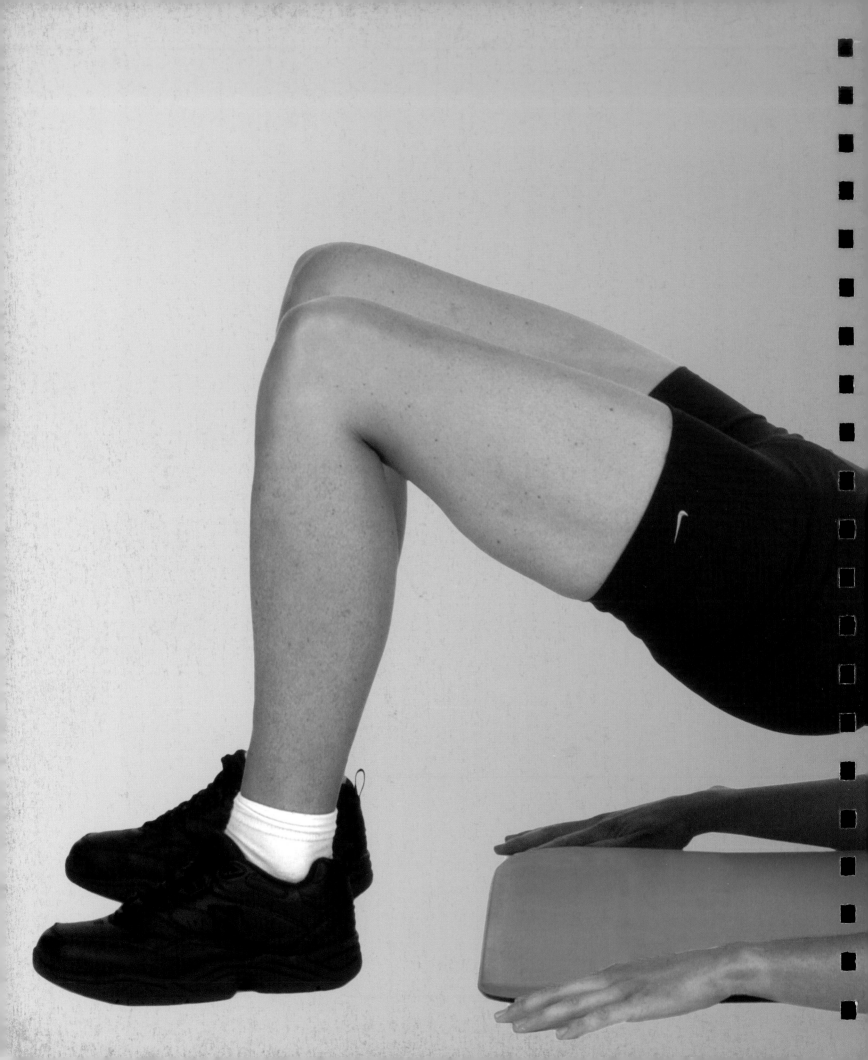

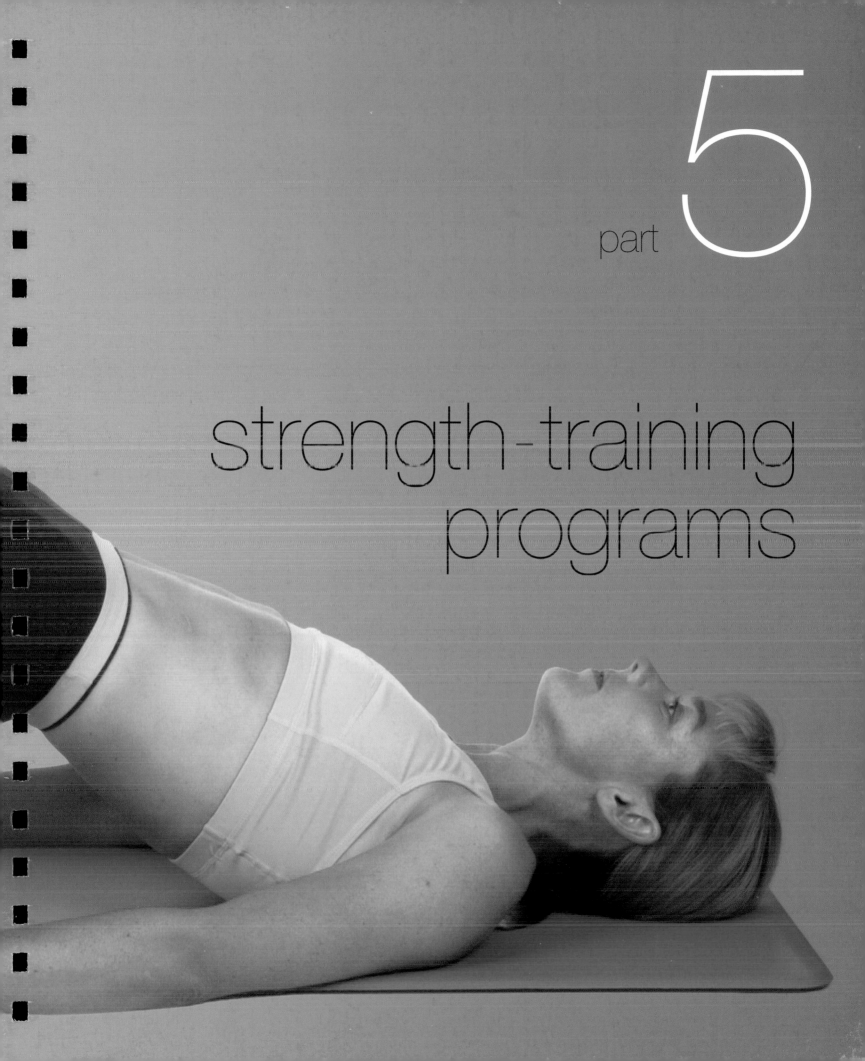

part 5

strength-training programs

devising your own programs

The programs on the following pages should be used as a basis for you to structure your own workout. How you decide to organize your program will depend on your level of ability and what you are trying to achieve through strength training.

If you are a beginner to strength training, your main goal should be to familiarize yourself with the exercises, learn the correct techniques, and get your untrained muscles accustomed to working out with added resistance.

As with any new system there is always a lot to learn and at first it may all seem a little overwhelming. As you work out, trying to remember the exercises, sets, reps, and training techniques will exhaust you before you've hardly begun. I would suggest using a training diary even up to advanced level.

Points to remember:
Sometimes I have varied the number of reps you need to do in a set (for example, 10–15 reps). Use this as a guide to increasing the intensity of an exercise as you progress through it. Start the first set with 10 reps, move on to 13 reps in the next set, and finish the last set with 15 reps.

The time indicated for each of the programs does not include any supplementary aerobic activity that may have been suggested.

strength-training diary

Below is an example of the type of information you need to record in your diary.

strength-training goal:

short-term	mid-term	ultimate goal

aerobic-training goal:

short-term	mid-term	ultimate goal

month: **date:**

strength-training exercise	sets	reps	goal for next workout

beginner level strength-training workout

This is an overall workout that should be attempted at least twice a week along with some aerobic exercises to see a benefit.

An example of a beginner weekly workout:

Monday—(whole body) weights/aerobics 20–30 minutes
Tuesday—rest
Wednesday—aerobics 30–40 minutes
Thursday—rest
Friday—(whole body) weights/aerobics 20–30 minutes
Weekend: Saturday—rest Sunday—rest

This is just a suggested guideline; how you ultimately decide to arrange your workout will depend on your fitness level, available time, and ultimate goal.

the workout

• Where possible, train in front of a mirror so that you can see exactly what you are doing.

• Workout time: around 1 hour (10-minute warm-up, 40 minutes training, 10-minute cool-down).

• It may take about 40 minutes to go through the exercises, though once you are familiar with them that time should reduce to 25–30 minutes.

• Try to do 3 minutes of aerobics between every two muscle groups that you work, to keep your heart rate up. For example: chest/shoulders—3 minutes of cardio; quads/hamstrings—3 minutes cardio; and so on.

• Warm up with light aerobic activity and gentle stretching.

• Use a comfortable weight that allows you a full range of movement. When starting off, it's best to try to arrange the exercises by muscle groups rather than jumping from one muscle to the next—you might get confused about which muscle you should be focusing on.

• Use your rest period between sets for stretching the particular muscle(s) you are working.

• Cool down by stretching your whole body (see stretching section on page 28).

Chest

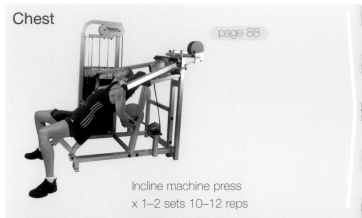

page 88

Incline machine press
x 1–2 sets 10–12 reps

Quads

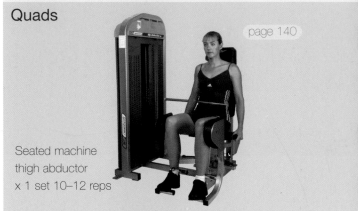

page 140

Seated machine thigh abductor
x 1 set 10–12 reps

Hamstrings

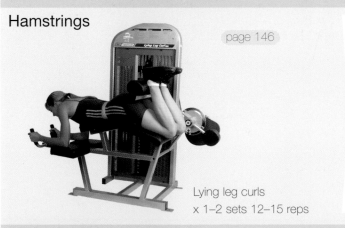

page 146

Lying leg curls
x 1–2 sets 12–15 reps

Triceps

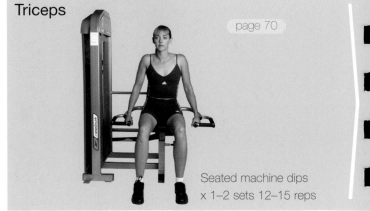

page 70

Seated machine dips
x 1–2 sets 12–15 reps

Shoulders

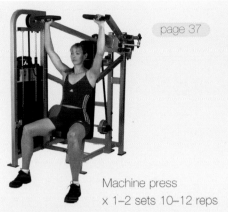

page 37

Machine press
x 1–2 sets 10–12 reps

Quads

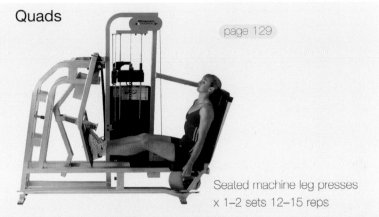

page 129

Seated machine leg presses
x 1–2 sets 12–15 reps

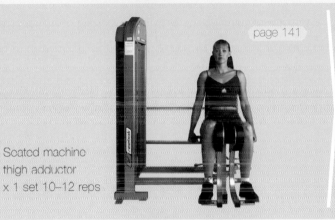

page 141

Seated machine
thigh adductor
x 1 set 10–12 reps

Glutes

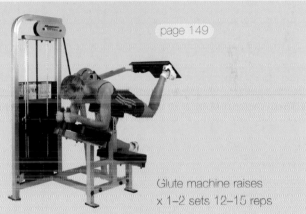

page 149

Glute machine raises
x 1–2 sets 12–15 reps

Back

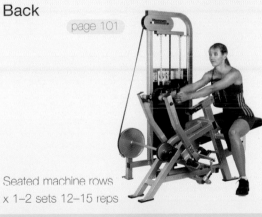

page 101

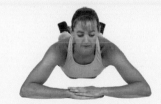

page 115

Seated machine rows
x 1–2 sets 12–15 reps

Floor back extensions
x 1–2 sets 12–15 reps

Biceps

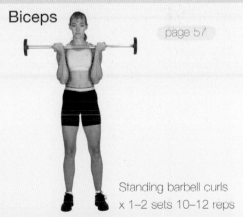

page 57

Standing barbell curls
x 1–2 sets 10–12 reps

Calves

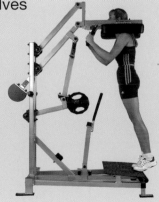

page 155

Standing machine calf raises
x 1–2 sets 12–15 reps

Abdominals

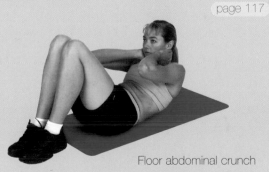

page 117

Floor abdominal crunch
x 1–2 sets 10–15 reps

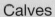

intermediate level strength-training workout

At this stage you should progressively be overloading your muscles and challenging them to work a little harder with each workout.

An example of an intermediate weekly workout:

Monday—weights/aerobics: chest/back/abs

Tuesday—rest

Wednesday—weights/aerobics: quads/hamstrings/glutes/calves

Thursday—rest

Friday—weights/aerobics: shoulders/biceps/triceps/abs

Weekend: Saturday—rest Sunday—aerobics

This is just a guideline; how you ultimately arrange your workout will depend on fitness level, time, and goals.

the workout

• Where possible, train in front of a mirror so that you can see exactly what you are doing.

• Workout time: 60–65 minutes (10-minute warm-up, 45 minutes training, 10-minute cool-down).

• Do your cardio training before or after training (30–40 minutes) or between every two muscle groups (5 minutes). Ultimately it will depend on your time restrictions in the gym.

• At this stage you will probably want to divide the different areas of the body into different training

sessions, so that you can work each area harder and more effectively. As you progress and slowly add more exercises, your workouts will become far too long if you try to train your whole body every time.

• Since there are more exercises per body part at this level, the workout should take a little longer.

• Warm up with light aerobic activity and gentle stretching.

• Cool down by stretching your whole body (see stretching section on page 28).

Use your rest period between sets for stretching the particular muscle(s) you are working.

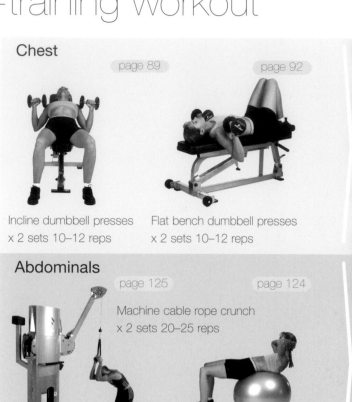

Chest

page 89   page 92

Incline dumbbell presses   Flat bench dumbbell presses
x 2 sets 10–12 reps   x 2 sets 10–12 reps

Abdominals

page 125   page 124

Machine cable rope crunch
x 2 sets 20–25 reps

Swiss-ball crunch
x 2 sets 20–30 reps

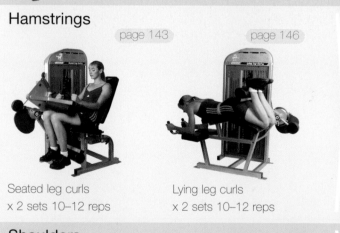

Hamstrings

page 143   page 146

Seated leg curls   Lying leg curls
x 2 sets 10–12 reps   x 2 sets 10–12 reps

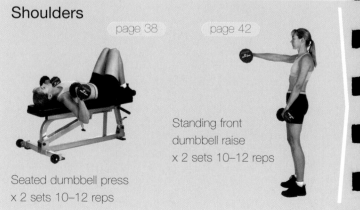

Shoulders

page 38   page 42

Standing front
dumbbell raise
x 2 sets 10–12 reps

Seated dumbbell press
x 2 sets 10–12 reps

Back

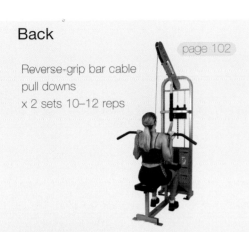

page 102

Reverse-grip bar cable pull downs
x 2 sets 10–12 reps

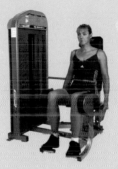

page 108

One-arm dumbbell rows
x 2 sets 10–12 reps

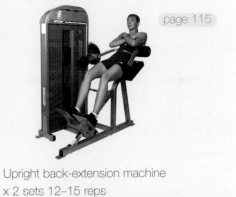

page 115

Upright back-extension machine
x 2 sets 12–15 reps

Quads

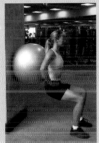

page 134

Swiss-ball squats
x 2 sets 15–20 reps

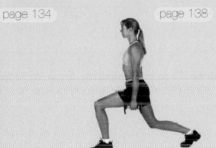

page 138

Stationary dumbbell forward lunges
x 2 sets 12–15 reps

page 140

Seated machine thigh abductor
x 2 sets 12–15 reps

page 141

Seated machine thigh adductor
x 2 sets 12–15 reps

Glutes

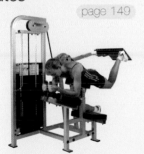

page 149

Glute machine raises
x 2 sets 12–15 reps

Calves

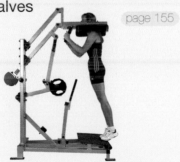

page 155

Standing machine calf raises
x 2 sets 12–15 reps

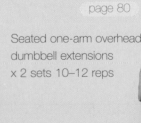

page 160

Seated calf raises
x 2 sets 12–15 reps

Biceps

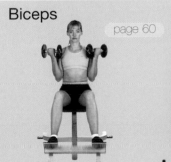

page 60

page 65

Standing one-arm dumbbell curl over bench
x 2 sets 10–12 reps

Seated dumbbell curls
x 2 sets 10–12 reps

Triceps

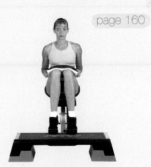

page 78

page 80

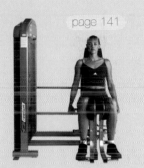

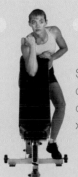

Seated one-arm overhead dumbbell extensions
x 2 sets 10–12 reps

Bench dumbbell kickbacks
x 2 sets 10–12 reps

strength-training program for seniors

The focus at this time in your life is strength and increased lean muscle mass.

An example of a weekly senior workout:

Monday—weights/aerobics: chest/back/lower back/abs

Tuesday—rest

Wednesday—rest

Thursday—weights/aerobics: quads/hamstrings/calves

Friday—rest

Weekend: Saturday—weights/aerobics: shoulders/biceps/triceps/abs

        Sunday—rest

If working out three times a week is too much, then keep it to one or two sessions a week until your strength and stamina have increased.

At this stage in your life it is especially important that you consult your physician before undertaking any new training program or system of exercise, particularly if you have any medical problems or injuries or are on any medication. You should take special care if you haven't exercised in many years or have never before followed a regular exercise routine. I urge you to seek advice from a qualified strength instructor or hire a personal trainer to guide you through your workouts.

Your program will be similar to that of a beginner, with more emphasis on strengthening the areas of the body that are more prone to injury as you get older, such as the lower back and hip region.

the workout

- Where possible, train in front of a mirror so that you can see exactly what you are doing.

- Workout time: around 1 hour (10-minute warm-up, 40 minutes training, 10-minute cool-down).

- It may take about 40 minutes for you to go through the exercises, though once you are familiar with them that time should reduce to 25–30 minutes.

- Try to complete 3 minutes of aerobics between every two muscle groups you work, to keep your heart rate up. For example: chest/shoulders—3 minutes of cardio—quads/hamstrings—3 minutes of cardio—and so on.

- Warm up with light aerobic activity and gentle stretching.

- Cool down by stretching your whole body (see stretching section on page 28).

Use a comfortable weight that allows you a full range of movement. When starting off, it's best to try to arrange the exercises by muscle groups rather than jumping from one muscle to the next—you might get confused about which muscle you should be focusing on.

Use your rest period between sets for stretching the particular muscle(s) you are working.

Chest

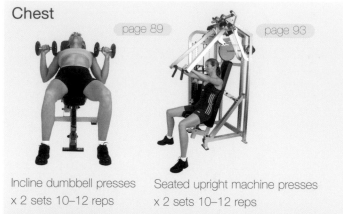

page 89   page 93

Incline dumbbell presses
x 2 sets 10–12 reps

Seated upright machine presses
x 2 sets 10–12 reps

Abdominals

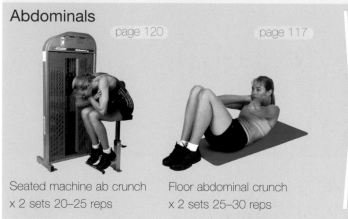

page 120   page 117

Seated machine ab crunch
x 2 sets 20–25 reps

Floor abdominal crunch
x 2 sets 25–30 reps

Quads

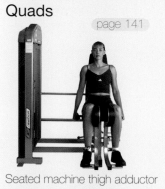

page 141

Seated machine thigh adductor
x 2 sets 10–12 reps

Hamstrings

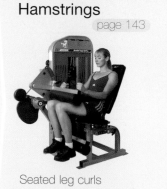

page 143

Seated leg curls
x 2 sets 10–12 reps

Shoulders

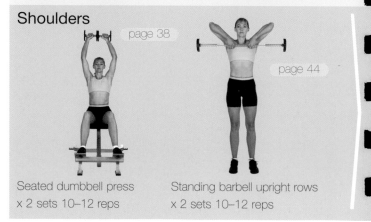

page 38

page 44

Seated dumbbell press
x 2 sets 10–12 reps

Standing barbell upright rows
x 2 sets 10–12 reps

Back

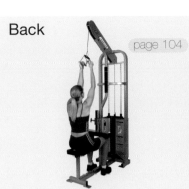
page 104

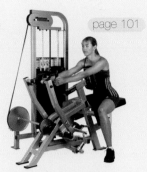
page 101

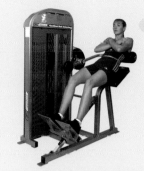
page 115

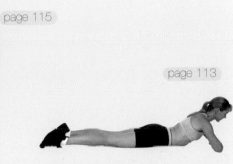
page 113

Seated V-bar pull downs
x 2 sets 10–12 reps

Seated machine rows
x 2 sets 10–12 reps

Upright back-extension machine
x 2 sets 10–12 reps

Floor back extensions
x 2 sets 12–15 reps

Quads

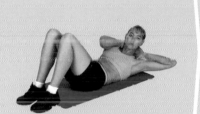
page 118

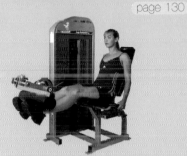
page 130

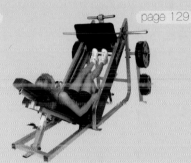
page 129

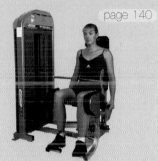
page 140

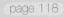

Cross-body oblique crunch
x 2 sets 15–20 reps

Seated machine leg extensions
x 2 sets 12–15 reps

Seated machine leg presses
x 2 sets 12–15 reps

Seated machine thigh abductor
x 2 sets 10–12 reps

Glutes

Calves

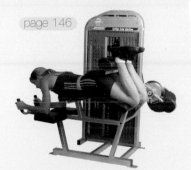
page 146

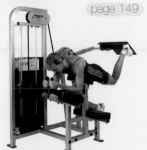
page 149

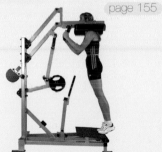
page 155

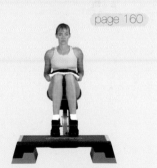
page 160

Lying leg curls
x 2 sets 10–12 reps

Glute machine raises
x 2 sets 12–15 reps

Standing machine calf raises
x 2 sets 10–12 reps

Seated calf raises
x 2 sets 10–12 reps

Biceps

Triceps

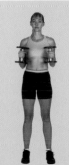
page 60

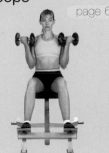
page 62

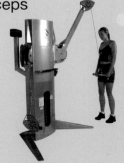
page 69

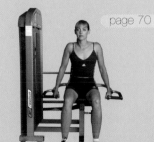
page 70

Seated dumbbell curls
x 2 sets 10–12 reps

Standing hammer dumbbell curls
x 2 sets 10–12 reps

Cable machine push downs
x 2 sets 10–12 reps

Seated machine dips
x 2 sets 10–12 reps

strength-training program for home training

The flexibility of home training allows anyone to maintain a regular training program.

An example of a weekly home training workout:

Monday—weights/aerobics: chest/back/lower back/abs

Tuesday—rest

Wednesday—rest

Thursday—weights/aerobics: quads/hamstrings/calves

Friday—rest

Weekend: Saturday—weights/aerobics: shoulders/biceps/triceps/abs

Sunday—rest

When training at home there is no need for any fancy equipment. All you need are a good pair of adjustable weights (the type that you can add extra weights to as you get stronger), an imagination (be creative with items you have at home that could be used instead of gym equipment), and the motivation to train instead of simply sitting in front of the television.

Depending on what stage you have reached with your training, whether you are a complete beginner or at intermediate level, I would suggest a minimum of two sessions per week (three if possible), along with three or four sessions of cardiovascular exercise. Obviously this will depend on what goals you have set for yourself and how much time you have available.

the workout

• Where possible, train in front of a mirror so that you can see exactly what you are doing.

• Workout time: around 1 hour (10-minute warm-up, 40 minutes training, 10-minute cool-down).

• It may take about 40 minutes to go through the exercises, though once you have become familiar with them that time should reduce to 25–30 minutes.

• The type of equipment, if any, that you have at home will determine what sort of aerobic training you are able do. If you

have nothing, I would suggest a good 30–40-minute power walk.

• Warm up with light aerobic activity and gentle stretching.

• Use a comfortable weight that allows you a full range of movement.

• Use your rest period between sets to stretch the particular muscle(s) you are working.

• Cool down by stretching your whole body (see stretching section on page 28).

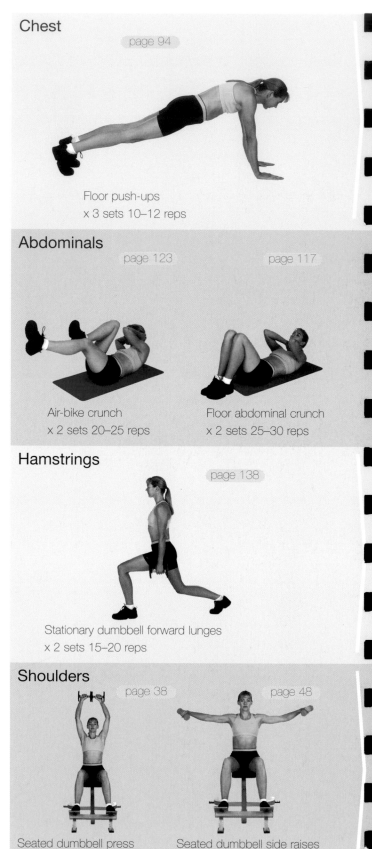

Chest
page 94

Floor push-ups
x 3 sets 10–12 reps

Abdominals
page 123   page 117

Air-bike crunch
x 2 sets 20–25 reps

Floor abdominal crunch
x 2 sets 25–30 reps

Hamstrings
page 138

Stationary dumbbell forward lunges
x 2 sets 15–20 reps

Shoulders
page 38   page 48

Seated dumbbell press
x 2 sets 10–12 reps

Seated dumbbell side raises
x 2 sets 10–12 reps

Back

page 108

page 113

page 114

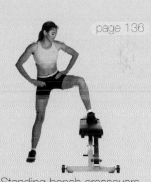

One-arm dumbbell rows
x 2 sets 10–12 reps

Floor back extensions
x 2 sets 10–12 reps

Opposite arm and leg back extensions
x 2 sets 12–15 reps

Quads

page 122

page 134

page 138

page 136

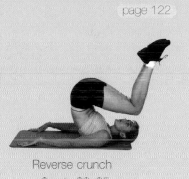

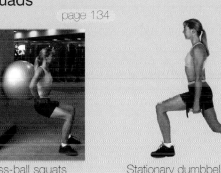

Reverse crunch
x 2 sets 20–25 reps

Swiss-ball squats
x 2 sets 15–20 reps

Stationary dumbbell forward lunges
x 2 sets 12–15 reps

Standing bench crossovers
x 2 sets 15–20 reps

Glutes

page 150

page 152

Calves

page 160

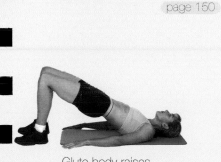

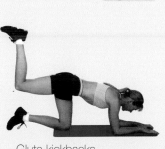

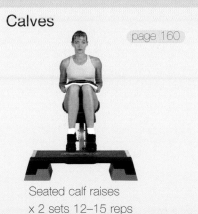

Glute body raises
x 2 sets 15–20 reps

Glute kickbacks
x 2 sets 15–20 reps

Seated calf raises
x 2 sets 12–15 reps

Biceps

page 60

page 66

Triceps

page 72

page 76

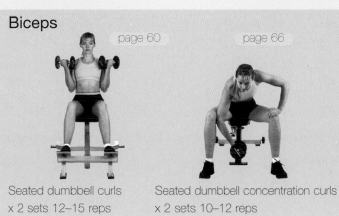

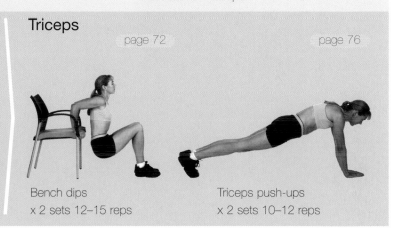

Seated dumbbell curls
x 2 sets 12–15 reps

Seated dumbbell concentration curls
x 2 sets 10–12 reps

Bench dips
x 2 sets 12–15 reps

Triceps push-ups
x 2 sets 10–12 reps

fat-loss and menopause training program

The hormonal changes of menopause mean that the problems of weight gain can become particularly relevant at this time of life.

An example of a weekly workout:

Monday—chest/shoulders/quads/hamstrings aerobics
Tuesday—aerobics 40 minutes–1 hour
Wednesday—rest
Thursday—aerobics 40 minutes–1 hour
Friday—back/biceps/triceps/calves/abs aerobics
Weekend: Saturday—rest Sunday—aerobics 40 minutes–1 hour

This is just a guideline; you should make appropriate changes depending on your individual level of fitness. If fat loss is your ultimate goal, it is important that you work toward this weekly training program or something similar.

Menopause and obesity have two things in common. Women who are going through menopause experience physical changes like hormonal changes that cause them to gain weight (weight gain can also be a side effect of taking medication such as HRT). At this time in a woman's life, losing weight can be very difficult because she is continually fighting against her ever-changing body.

Overweight women often have issues similar to those of women going through menopause. Losing weight can be an uphill battle, as you are fighting against physical changes in the body from the onset of being overweight as well as trying to overcome psychological issues as to why you may have become overweight in the first place.

This program has a stronger emphasis on aerobic training to help increase your metabolism and encourage you to burn as many calories as possible while at rest as well as while active, with some high-repetition strength-training compound exercises that will work as many muscle groups as possible to increase lean muscle mass and burn even more calories.

the workout

• Where possible, train in front of a mirror so that you can see exactly what you are doing.

• Workout time: around 1 hour (not including aerobic activity) (10-minute warm-up, 1 hour training, 10-minute cool-down).

• Warm up with light aerobic activity and gentle stretching.

• Use a comfortable weight that allows you a full range of movement.

• Use your rest period between sets to stretch the particular muscle(s) you are working.

• Cool down by stretching your whole body (see stretching section on page 28).

Chest

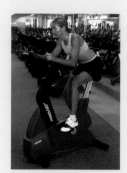

10 minutes exercise bike

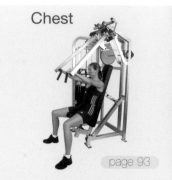

page 93

Seated upright machine presses x 2 sets 15–18 reps

Quads

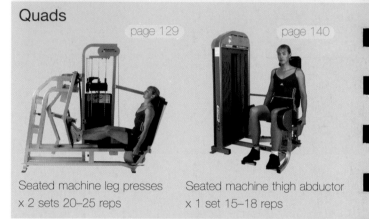

page 129   page 140

Seated machine leg presses x 2 sets 20–25 reps

Seated machine thigh abductor x 1 set 15–18 reps

Back

page 102

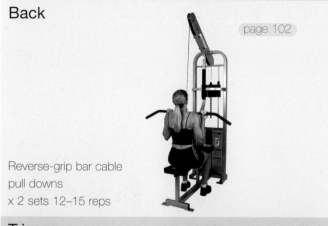

Reverse-grip bar cable pull downs x 2 sets 12–15 reps

Triceps

page 70

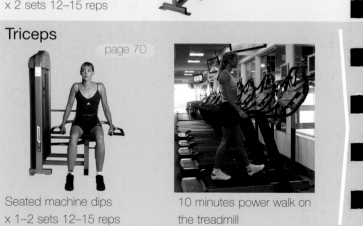

Seated machine dips x 1–2 sets 12–15 reps

10 minutes power walk on the treadmill

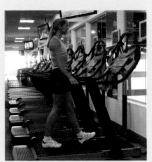

10 minutes power walk
on the treadmill

Shoulders

page 37

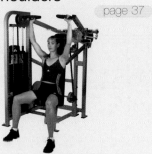

Machine press (military press)
x 2 sets 15–18 reps

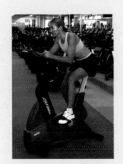

10 minutes exercise bike

page 141

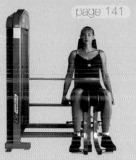

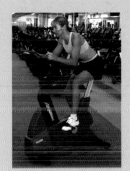

Seated machine thigh adductor
x 1 set 15–18 reps

10 minutes exercise bike

Hamstrings

page 143

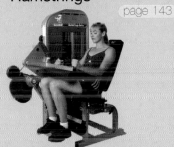

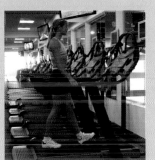

Seated leg curls
x 2 sets 16–20 reps

10 minutes power walk
on the treadmill

page 113

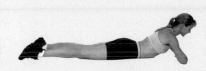

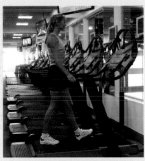

Floor back extensions
x 1–2 sets 12–15 reps

10 minutes power walk
on the treadmill

Biceps

page 67

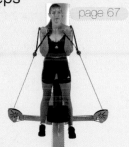

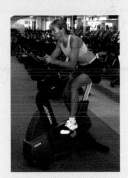

Standing two-arm cable curls
x 1–2 sets 12–15 reps

10 minutes exercise bike

Calves

page 155

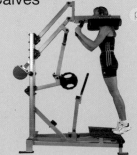

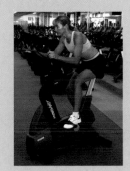

Standing machine calf raises
x 1–2 sets 15–18 reps

10 minutes exercise bike

Abdominals

page 117

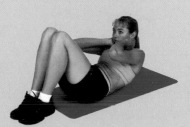

Floor abdominal crunch
x 1–2 sets 20–25 reps

training during pregnancy

Consult with your physician and train with a qualified strength instructor who is experienced in working with pregnant women. Since your limbs tend to be softer and more supple at this time, you are more prone to injury.

An example of a training workout while pregnant:

Monday—(whole body) weights/aerobics

Tuesday—rest

Wednesday—aerobics 30–40 minutes

Thursday—rest

Friday—(whole body) weights/aerobics

Weekend: Saturday—rest Sunday—rest

This is just a guideline; how you ultimately arrange your individual workout will depend on your fitness level, time available, and personal goals. *Be sure to consult with your doctor before starting a training program.*

Many years ago it was believed that when a woman was pregnant she should cease all exercise for the full nine months; too much activity was thought to be unhealthy for the woman and the unborn child. Nowadays we know better—keeping fit and staying active even while pregnant is essential for the health of the mother and her unborn child, and it can also make childbirth easier and recovery faster.

From the start of your pregnancy right up until you give birth, it is important to continually adjust your exercise program as your body changes. The size of your ever-growing belly will make some exercises, like crunches, impossible to do, even at a fairly early stage. At certain stages of this program, I have included extra exercises for specific parts of the body such as the back. The additional weight of the baby means that it is vital for you to keep the surrounding muscle groups (such as the back and legs) as strong as possible in order for them to be able to cope effectively with the sudden extra weight.

the workout

• Where possible, train in front of a mirror so that you can see exactly what you are doing.

• Workout time: around 1 hour (10-minute warm-up, 40 minutes training, 10-minute cool-down).

• It may take about 40 minutes to go through the exercises, though once you are familiar with them that time should reduce to 25–30 minutes.

• Try to do 3 minutes of aerobics between every two muscle groups you work, to keep your heart rate up. For example: chest/shoulders—3 minutes of cardio—quads/hamstrings—3 minutes cardio—and so on.

• Warm up with light aerobic activity and gentle stretching.

• Use a comfortable weight that allows you a full range of movement.

• Use your rest period between sets to stretch the particular muscle(s) you are working.

• Cool down by stretching your whole body (see stretching section on page 28).

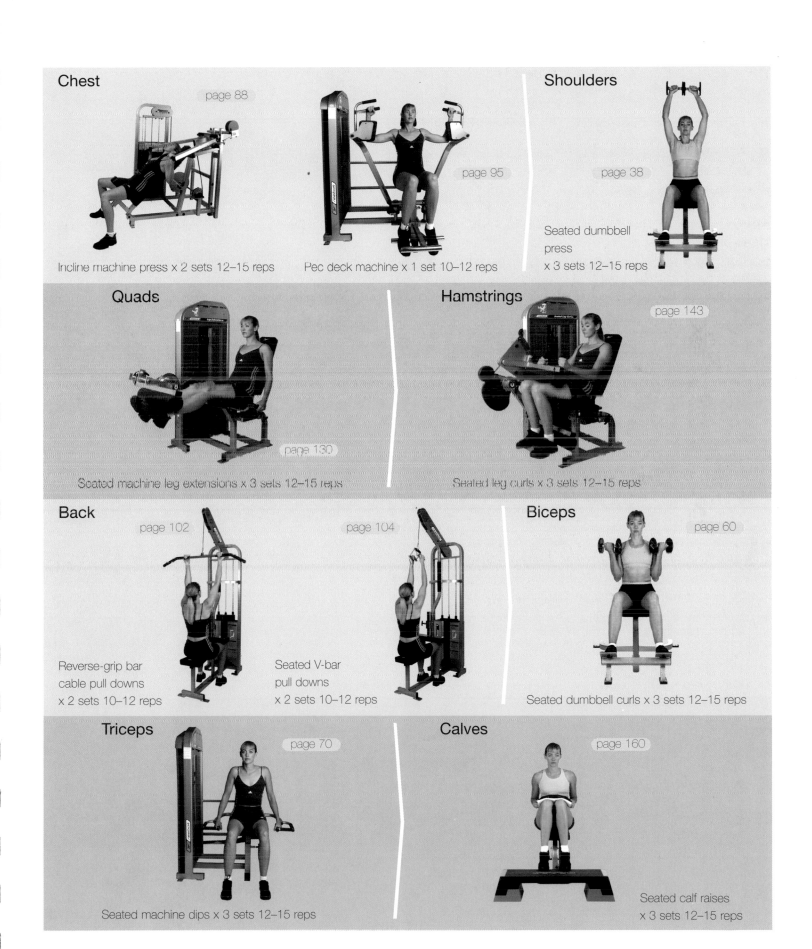

Chest

page 88

page 95

Incline machine press x 2 sets 12–15 reps

Pec deck machine x 1 set 10–12 reps

Shoulders

page 38

Seated dumbbell
press
x 3 sets 12–15 reps

Quads

page 130

Seated machine leg extensions x 3 sets 12–15 reps

Hamstrings

page 143

Seated leg curls x 3 sets 12–15 reps

Back

page 102

page 104

Reverse-grip bar
cable pull downs
x 2 sets 10–12 reps

Seated V-bar
pull downs
x 2 sets 10–12 reps

Biceps

page 60

Seated dumbbell curls x 3 sets 12–15 reps

Triceps

page 70

Seated machine dips x 3 sets 12–15 reps

Calves

page 160

Seated calf raises
x 3 sets 12–15 reps

muscular size–building program

The effectiveness of this program will depend very much on your body type and ability to increase muscle mass.

An example of a muscular size weekly workout:

Monday—(whole body) weights

Tuesday—rest

Wednesday—aerobics 30–40 minutes

Thursday—rest

Friday—(whole body) weights

Weekend: Saturday—rest Sunday—rest

This is just a guideline; how you choose to ultimately arrange your workout will depend on how much muscular size you need to gain as well as the time you have available and your personal goals.

If you are lucky enough to be an ectomorph body type with long limbs, a fast metabolism, and little to no body fat, gaining muscular size to fill out your body can be an uphill battle. Although it is not impossible for you to obtain some sort of muscular size, it will never be to the same extent as that of a mesomorph.

If you are an ectomorph it is essential that you pay careful attention to diet and nutrition as you may well burn calories faster than you can eat. It may be a good idea to supplement your diet with a weight-gain bodybuilding drink. Weight-gain supplements add the extra calories needed to put on weight, as it can be virtually impossible to eat the amount of calories that you may need to increase your lean muscle mass. You may find it best to consult a qualified strength instructor or nutritionist to advise you on your diet and supplement needs.

The workout outlined below has a stronger emphasis on strength training than aerobic exercise. Although it is necessary to maintain your fitness, if you do more aerobic exercise than suggested here, you will hamper gaining any real size, because aerobic training will increase your already fast metabolism.

the workout

• Where possible, train in front of a mirror so that you can see exactly what you are doing.

• Workout time: around 1 hour (10-minute warm-up, 40 minutes training, 10-minute cool-down).

• It may take about 40 minutes to go through the exercises, though once you are familiar with them that time should reduce to 25–30 minutes.

• Warm up with light aerobic activity and gentle stretching.

• Use a comfortable weight that allows you a full range of movement.

• Use your rest period between sets to stretch the particular muscle(s) you are working.

• Cool down by stretching your whole body (see stretching section on page 28).

Chest

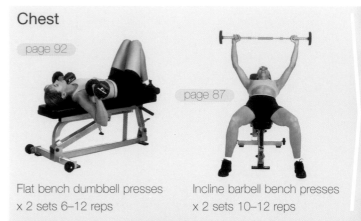

Flat bench dumbbell presses x 2 sets 6–12 reps

Incline barbell bench presses x 2 sets 10–12 reps

page 92

page 87

Quads

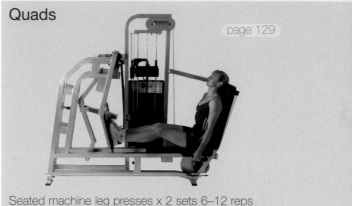

page 129

Seated machine leg presses x 2 sets 6–12 reps

Back

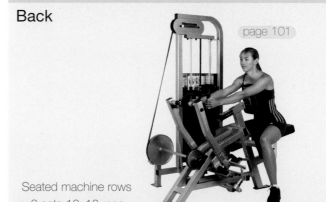

page 101

Seated machine rows x 3 sets 10–12 reps

Triceps

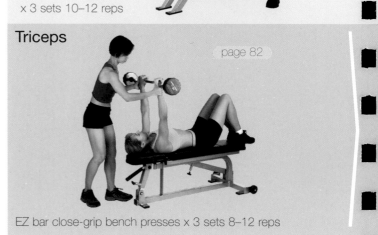

page 82

EZ bar close-grip bench presses x 3 sets 8–12 reps

Shoulders

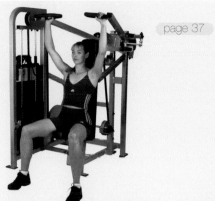

page 37

Machine press
(military press)
x 2 sets 10–12 reps

page 44

Standing barbell upright rows
x 2 sets 10–12 reps

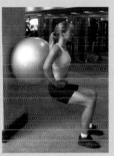

page 134

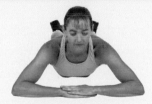

Swiss-ball squats
x 2 sets 10–12 reps

Hamstrings

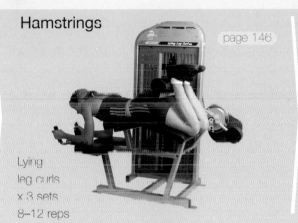

page 146

Lying
leg curls
x 3 sets
8–12 reps

Glutes

page 149

Glute machine raises
x 3 sets 12–15 reps

page 113

Floor back extensions
x 2 sets 10–12 reps

Biceps

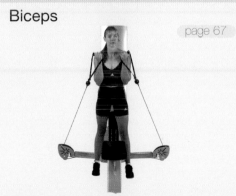

page 67

page 58

Standing two-arm cable curls x 2 sets 8–10 reps   Standing dumbbell curls x 2 sets 8–10 reps

Calves

page 155

Standing machine calf raises
x 2 sets 12–15 reps

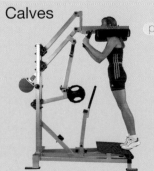

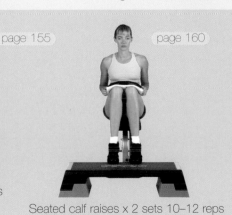

page 160

Seated calf raises x 2 sets 10–12 reps

Abdominals

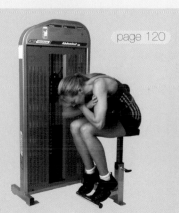

page 120

Seated machine
abdominal crunch
x 3 sets 15–20 reps

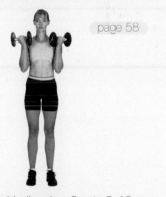

shape and tone strength-training program

This routine consists of high reps, as the emphasis is on shaping your muscles rather than building muscle.

An example of a shape and tone weekly workout:

Monday—chest/back/shoulders/abs aerobics

Tuesday—rest

Wednesday—quads/hamstrings/glutes aerobics

Thursday—rest

Friday—biceps/triceps/calves/abs aerobics

Weekend: Saturday—rest Sunday—aerobics 30–40 minutes

This is just a guideline; how you ultimately arrange your workout will depend on how much you need to shape and tone your physique, the time you have available, and your personal goals.

If there were only two little words in the vocabulary of any woman starting out in strength training they would be "shape" and "tone." Whoever I train and wherever I am in the world discussing strength training, these seem to be the first words to come out of every woman's mouth. I must confess that even in my own training this is what I'm constantly striving for.

the workout

• Where possible, train in front of a mirror so that you can see exactly what you are doing.

• Workout time: around 1 hour (10-minute warm-up, 40 minutes training, 10-minute cool-down).

• You should do at least 30–40 minutes of cardio either before or after your workout, using an exercise bike, treadmill, stair machine, or rowing machine.

• Warm up with light aerobic activity and gentle stretching.

• Use weights that allow you a full range of movement.

• Use your rest period between sets to stretch the particular muscle(s) that you are working.

• Cool down by stretching your whole body (see stretching section on page 28).

Chest

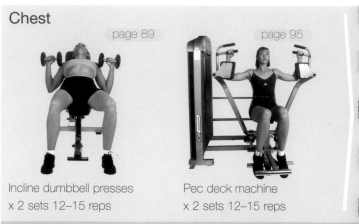

page 89   page 95

Incline dumbbell presses
x 2 sets 12–15 reps

Pec deck machine
x 2 sets 12–15 reps

Shoulders

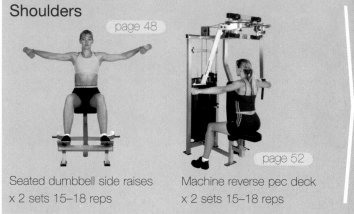

page 48   page 52

Seated dumbbell side raises
x 2 sets 15–18 reps

Machine reverse pec deck
x 2 sets 15–18 reps

Quads

page 136   page 140

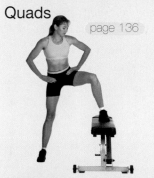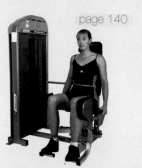

Standing bench crossovers
x 2 sets 15–20 reps

Seated machine thigh abductor
x 3 sets 15–20 reps

Biceps

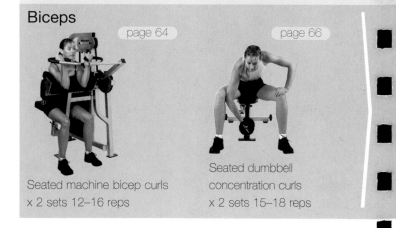

page 64   page 66

Seated machine bicep curls
x 2 sets 12–16 reps

Seated dumbbell
concentration curls
x 2 sets 15–18 reps

Back

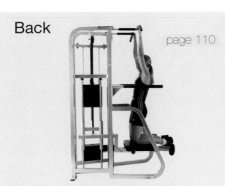
page 110

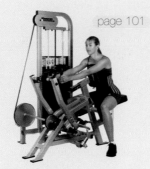
page 101

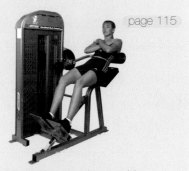
page 115

Supported machine chin-ups
x 2 sets 12–15 reps

Seated machine rows
x 2 sets 12–15 reps

Upright back-extension machine
x 2 sets 12–15 reps

Abdominals

page 118

page 124

page 122

Quads

page 138

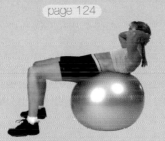

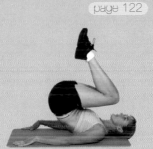

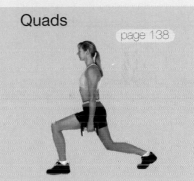

Cross-body oblique crunch
x 2 sets 25–30 reps

Swiss ball crunch
x 2 sets 20–30 reps
(alternate with floor crunch)

Reverse crunch
x 2 sets 20–30 reps

Stationary dumbbell forward lunges
x 2 sets 20–25 reps

Hamstrings
Glutes

page 141

page 146

page 143

page 149

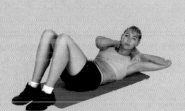

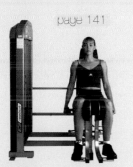

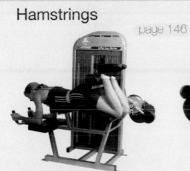

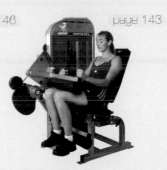

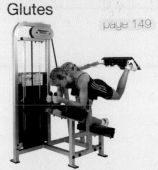

Seated machine thigh adductor
x 3 sets 15–20 reps

Lying leg curls
x 2 sets 15–16 reps

Seated leg curls
x 2 sets 15–16 reps

Glute machine raises
x 3 sets 12–18 reps

Triceps
Calves

page 72

page 69

page 155

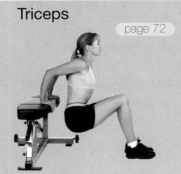

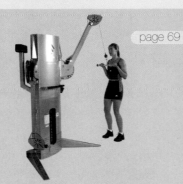

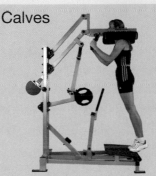

Bench dips
x 2 sets 15–18 reps

Cable machine push downs
x 2 sets 12–16 reps

Standing machine calf raises
x 2 sets 12–15 reps

glossary of strength-training terms

Though there are hundreds of strength-training terms, here I have listed the essential terms that a beginner or intermediate strength trainer will come across.

Abduction, abductor Abduction is movement away from the center of the body. An abductor is a muscle whose contraction results in this movement.

Adduction, adductor Adduction is movement toward the center of the body. An adductor is a muscle whose contraction results in this movement.

Aerobics or aerobic exercise Exercise using oxygen for energy production. In strength training, aerobic exercise is normally used to promote the loss of body fat.

Anabolic steroids A term usually heard in bodybuilding; something that is "anabolic" in nature is said to encourage the growth of new muscle tissue. The word "anabolic" is often used with the term "steroid" but the two terms have separate and distinct meanings. Good nutrition, enough protein, and other legal substances also promote and support the growth of muscle tissue and therefore, are also anabolic in nature.

Anaerobic exercise Explosive, short bursts of exercise that don't require oxygen as an energy source. This type of training can be sustained only for short periods of time through lack of oxygen production.

Barbell Basic strength-training equipment along with dumbbells. A straight or slightly curved bar either already with weights on the ends or designed to have them placed manually on the ends. A typical barbell is about one inch to one-and-an-eighth inches in diameter and five to seven feet long.

Basic (basal) metabolic rate The rate at which the body burns calories at rest (when not exercising), typically measured in calories per day.

Bicep A large two-headed muscle at the front of the upper arm that bends the forearm toward the shoulders. The biceps function in pulling and curling movements.

Bodybuilder Someone who uses strength training to improve their body and overall well-being. Only a fraction of all bodybuilders are competitive.

Body composition An analysis of the proportions of fat, muscle, and bone making up the body. Usually expressed as percent of body fat and percent of lean body mass (LBM).

Bulking up An old term used for gaining weight by adding both fat and muscle by eating as much as you can while training as hard as possible.

Burn A burning sensation felt in the specific muscle or muscles when training the muscle to exhaustion. This reaction is due to the presence of lactic acid in the tissues, a waste product of glucose metabolism during intense exercise. A trainer welcomes the burn, as the degree of burn endured indicates the level of muscle overload achieved, a key factor in muscle building.

Calories Used to describe the energy value of nutrients. Calorie beginning with a capital "C" is the common term for kilocalorie (kcal), while calorie with a lowercase "c" is one thousandth of a kilocalorie.

Cardio Pertaining to activity that raises the resting heart rate. This is strength-training jargon for moderate to intense aerobic activity.

Cardiovascular fitness (see aerobics) The ability of the heart to pump oxygen to the organs and the ability of the organs to use the oxygen. The fitter you are, the better your aerobic system.

Collars, weight collars Any kind of protective sleeve that can be slipped over the end of a weight bar after the plates have been put on and then tightened to hold the plates securely and safely on the bar; they keep the plates from slipping off the end of the bar, changing position, or moving during exercising.

Compound exercises These are exercises that work the smaller, larger, and surrounding muscle groups. They are often used for mass gain. An example of a compound exercise is the machine leg press.

Concentric contraction Shortening of a muscle due to muscle contraction. Also known as the positive phase or positive contraction. For example, pulling the weight up toward your shoulders in a biceps curl movement.

Deltoid or delt A large, three-part muscle (front, side, and rear deltoid) of the shoulder that moves the arms away from the body.

Dehydration A condition resulting from the excessive loss of body water. It can lead to fainting.

Dumbbell Short-handled basic weight equipment that usually comes in matching pairs.

Eccentric contraction Lengthening of a muscle while under the tension of resistance. Also known as the negative phase or negative contraction. For example, lowering the weight in a biceps curl back down toward your thighs.

Extension The straightening of a simple joint such as the knee that makes your leg straight, as in the leg extension.

EZ curl bar or bent bar A specially bent barbell that places less strain on your wrists.

Flow A strength-training term referring to smooth, continuous movements from exercise to exercise without any interruption in focus.

Focus A mental process used when training to concentrate on the exercise and the muscle that you are working.

Full range of motion The total action of muscle(s) and the associated joint(s) from lifting the weight from start to finish fully.

Getting ripped Bodybuilding slang for achieving extreme definition and having the appearance of little to no fat through severe dieting. Usually associated with competitive bodybuilders.

Glucose Blood sugar. The broken down and transportable form of carbohydrate that fuels the cells. Also known as dextrose, grape sugar, or corn sugar.

Gluteus maximus (glutes, butt, bottom, rear) The outermost muscle of the three glutei found in each of the human buttocks.

Glycogen Sugar derived from animal starch. Glycogen is stored in the liver where it's changed into glucose and used as energy.

Grip, false (thumbless grip) A style of grip most commonly used in the reverse-grip bar cable pull downs in which the thumb remains against the side of the palm rather than wrapping around the bar. Palms should face you.

Grip, neutral (thumbs on grip) If your palms are facing toward you, you are using a neutral grip and your thumbs are over the bar rather than under it.

Grip, pronated A style of grip in which your palms face the floor while holding a weight.

Grip, supinated A style of grip in which your palms face you while holding a weight.

Hamstring or ham Short for hamstring muscle, any of three muscles at the back of the thigh that function to flex and rotate the leg and extend the thigh.

High reps Used in strength training where high repetitions (usually above twelve) of given exercises are performed for specific purposes (exercise practice, muscle warm-up, injury repair, muscularity, sport conditioning, weight loss).

Hypermobile Describes joints that are unusually mobile, especially those in pregnant women (during pregnancy, the hormone relaxin softens ligaments to aid childbirth).

Isolation The exercising of one specific muscle exclusively, without the involvement of other muscles.

Lactic acid A waste product of glucose and glycogen metabolism produced in the muscles during the hard work of exercise. Its existence is accompanied by muscle fatigue and a burning sensation.

Latissimus dorsi or lats Large muscles of the back that are chiefly responsible for the V shape noticed in male and female bodybuilders.

Lean body mass (LBM) Your body mass, excluding fat mass. Sixty to 70 percent of your LBM is water.

Lean body weight Your body weight, excluding fat.

Low reps A type of training that involves performing low repetitions (less than six) for specific effects in training (muscle mass, bulk, weight gain, power).

Mass Sheer size of muscle.

Obesity Being severely overweight. A body fat percentage exceeding 30.

Overtraining A state that occurs when you work out too often, resulting in the breaking of muscles faster than the body can rebuild them and rest. This can result in a lowered immune system and lead to illness and injuries.

Pace In strength training, a term that refers to the speed at which one trains. Pace will vary with personality, purpose, mood, or external factors.

Pectorals or pecs Broad fan-shaped muscles across the chest. Their prime function is abducting the arms—moving the arms across the chest.

Poundage The amount of weight or resistance (in pounds) used in strength training.

Pump Strength-training slang referring to the enlarged and tightened sensation the trainer experiences within the working muscle resulting from blood engorgement.

Pumping iron Originating in the 1950s, slang for lifting weights. The term was made famous by the 1977 documentary *Pumping Iron*.

Quadricep or quad A major four-part muscle in the front thigh primarily engaged in extending the leg at the knee.

Repetition or rep One complete movement of an exercise.

Rhythm A term used to describe the sensation of flow and pace in sport performance. The strength trainer's rhythm of training is achieved when functions are efficient and unimpeded.

Ripped A condition of extremely low body fat that can only be held for a short period of time. Describes the appearance of "rips" in the muscles through the skin. This term is usually associated with competitive bodybuilders.

Routine The sum of reps, sets, and exercises in any given workout.

Set Prescribed number of repetitions of any given exercise. Example: one set of eight repetitions.

Six-pack Defined abdominal muscles where you see six bulges (three per side) visible through the skin. The level of body fat needed to see all six varies between individuals. The lower muscles (near the pelvic region) usually require the lowest body fat levels to bring them out.

Split workout A workout divided into two or more parts, thereby allowing different muscle groups to be worked at different times of the day (morning and evening) or on different days.

Spot Provide assistance to someone who is working out and either is using heavy weight or needs assistance and guidance while training.

Spotter The person who spots.

Strength instructor (personal trainer) A qualified instructor who works one-on-one with you to teach, motivate, inspire, and assist in all aspects of your training.

Superset Two exercises performed alternately; one exercise followed by a second exercise before resting; for instance, a biceps curl followed by a triceps extension is one superset.

Tendinitis Inflammation of a tendon, the tough band of connective tissue that connects muscle to bone. This is a common problem among athletes who train too hard or overtrain and allow themselves to get out of condition on occasion. Tendons, unfortunately, take a long time to heal.

Tendon A band of strong and fibrous (collagenous) tissue, often cordlike in appearance, that connects muscles to bones and other structures.

Torso In bodybuilding, the trunk and midsection muscles: abdominals, obliques, erectors, intercostals.

Tricep or tri The muscle on the back of the upper arm, which is used primarily for extending the elbow.

Uptake Absorption of a substance, especially into a cell or tissue. For example, uptake of nutrients into the muscle.

V-taper Slang for a strength trainer who has a wide V-shaped back, broad shoulders, and small waist. Also used to describe what can be achieved through strength training.

Vascularity The visibility of veins on a strength trainer due to low body fat and genetics.

Volume In bodybuilding, the total number of sets and reps completed in a workout.

Washboard abs "Ripped" abdominal muscles—extremely low in body fat. The rectus abdominals are visibly seen, with the appearance of a washboard.

Working in The practice of cooperatively working with someone who is using a particular piece of equipment on the gym floor that you want to use, too.

Workout A collection of exercises, usually performed either at the gym or in your home. Also used to describe one complete exercise session.

resources

strength-training and fitness organizations

International Fitness Association
12472 Lake Underhill Road, #341
Orlando, Florida 32828
Tel: 800-227-1976 or 407-579-8610

National Association for Health and Fitness (NAHF)
c/o New York State Physical Activity Coalition
65 Niagara Square, Room 607
Buffalo, NY 14202
Tel: 716-583-0521
Fax: 716-851-4309
E-mail: NAHF@hotmail.com

National Gym Association, Inc.
P.O. Box 970579
Coconut Creek, Fl 33097-0579
Tel: 954-344-8410
Fax: 954-344-8412
E-mail: Info@nationalgym.com (general)
  Hr@nationalgym.com (human resources)
  Pr@nationalgym.com (public relations)
  Sales@nationalgym.com (sales)

National Strength & Conditioning Association
4575 Galley End
Suite 400B
Colorado Springs, CO 80915
Tel: 719-632-6722
Fax: 719-632-6367
Toll-free: 800-815-6826
National Headquarters: nsca@nsca-lift.org

American Alliance for Health, Physical Education, Recreation & Dance
1900 Association Dr.
Reston, VA 20191-1598
Tel: 800-213-7193

American Association for Active Lifestyles	x430
American Association for Health Education	x437
American Association for Leisure and Recreation	x472
Convention Department	x465
Districts	x416
Membership Department	x490
National Association for Girls and Women in Sport	x453
National Association for Sport and Physical Education	x410
National Dance Association	x464

American Society of Exercise Physiologists (ASEP)
National Office
c/o Dr. Tommy Boone
Department of Exercise Physiology
The College of St. Scholastica
1200 Kenwood Avenue
Duluth, MN 55811
Tel: 218 723 6297
E-mail: tboone2@css.edu

International Federation of BodyBuilders (IFBB)
2875 Bates Road
Montreal, Quebec, Canada H3S 1B7
Tel: 514-731-3783
Fax: 514-731-7082
E-mail: info@ifbb.com

useful Web sites

For further information or to contact the author of this book please
go to: **www.amazinlethi.com**

www.fitnessonline.com
Fitness information and services

www.womenfitness.net
Women's fitness

www.association-of-womens-fitness.org
Women's fitness

www.health-information-resource.com
Health and fitness resources

www.netsweat.com
Fitness and equipment resources

www.ballyfitness.com
Bally gyms

www.crunch.com
Crunch gym locations in major cities including New York, Chicago, Miami, Los Angeles, and San Francisco.

www.fitnessusa.com
Provides personal trainers, nutritional guidance, aerobic classes, resistance exercise, toning, and conditioning.

www.goldsgym.com
Gold's gyms

www.ladyofamerica.com
Women-only health and fitness clubs with international locations.

www.lafitness.com
LA Fitness gyms

www.livingwell.com
LivingWell gyms

www.24hourfitness.com
24 Hour Fitness gyms

www.virginactive.com/us/
Virgin Active gyms

www.ymca.net
Official site for the community service organization working to meet the health and social service needs of men, women, and children.

www.fitnesszone.com/gyms
Health & Fitness Gym Finder

www.wnbf.net
Official World Natural Bodybuilding Federation Web site

www.nabba.com
National Amateur Bodybuilders Association (NABBA)

useful books

Sculpting Her Body Perfect
Brad Schoenfeld and Kiana Tom (Foreword)
Human Kinetics, 1999
A progressive program of resistance exercises to strengthen and sculpt the physique.

A Woman's Book of Strength
Karen Andes
Perigree, 1995
A combination of diet, exercise, and relaxation techniques to promote both inner and outer strength.

Strength Training for Women Only: How to Double Your Strength in Only Six Weeks
Joseph F. Mullen
Universe.com, 2003
A time-efficient and productive approach to getting into shape, based on years of scientific research.

Strength Training for Women
Willye White (Foreword), James A. Peterson, Cedric X. Bryant, and Susan L. Peterson
Human Kinetics, 1995
A practical guide designed especially for women who want specific training programs and exercises involving a variety of equipment.

Women's Strength Training Anatomy
Frederic Delavier
Human Kinetics, 2003
Exercises for shaping and toning buttocks, abs, legs, and back are accompanied by full-color, detailed anatomical drawings.

The Body Sculpting Bible for Women
James Villepigue and Hugo A. Rivera
Hatherleigh Press, 2002
A fitness manual that aims to give women a defined, healthy figure through strength training and proper diet.

Strength Training for Beginners
Susie Dinan and Joan Bassey
HarperResource, 2003
A program of simple exercises, all of which can be performed at home, designed for women thirty-five and up to get toned and feel energized.

Basic Weight Training for Men and Women
Thomas D. Fahey
McGraw-Hill, 1999
A practical manual with helpful diagrams that describes how to develop a personalized strength-training program.

The Aerobics Program for Total Well-Being
Kenneth H. Cooper
Bantam Books, 1991
Combines advice on exercise, nutrition, and emotional well-being, and encourages the reader to design his/her own weekly exercise program.

Keep Moving!: Fitness Through Aerobics and Step
by Esther Pryor, Minda Goodman Kraines
McGraw Hill, 2000
Illustrations show the basic movements of step and floor aerobics, while the text discusses how to master difficult moves and avoid injury.

The Optimum Nutrition Bible: The Book You Have to Read if You Care About Your Health
Patrick Holford
Crossing Press, 1998
A nutrition guide explaining how to give yourself the best possible intake of nutrients, thereby increasing your energy and fitness levels.

An Introduction to Nutrition and Metabolism
David A. Bender
Taylor & Francis, 2002
Aims to explain the relationship between diet and health, nutrition and metabolism, with the help of clear diagrams.

index